I0841264

The Truth About... Vol. 6 – Controlling Cholesterol without Drugs
By B. K. Robinson
Copyright 2018© ALL RIGHTS RESERVED

READ THIS FIRST!
I hate writing introductions because I rarely read them. This is usually because the author tries to include some autobiographical anecdote about something that happened to him or her in childhood and quite frankly; I am just not interested. However, this is a "truth about" book in a series of them, so I try to pack it with important information from cover to cover.

I'm no doctor, nor do I have any kind of degree related to the subject matter of this book. As such you are welcome to judge me accordingly but, a whole lot of people have changed the world and the way you live and they did not have degrees either. So I recommend you read this booklet first, before you judge me and I think you will see that a person does not need a degree to be smart, hard working, well informed, and indeed an expert in their field.

That paragraph was lifted directly from the previous books in the series but I feel obligated to start by telling you the TRUTH about myself: I am NOT claiming to be some arrogant self-aggrandizing jackass with a wall full of diplomas. I am claiming to be a bewildered consumer like most people who just got tired of being so bewildered and went on a mission to find the TRUTH about nutrition (amongst many other topics for coming "truth about" books.)

One of the things that really got to me was the wide ocean of buzz words in the field of medicine and health. We all have heard of cholesterol but what is it and what does it do? This book will explain what it is, what it does, why it is in the blood, and what exactly "bad or high cholesterol" means and most importantly: how to take control of it and get those levels down and in the correct proportions which is really the central concern with cholesterol.

And our problems are only beginning with the invention of fake foods like soda pop that has NOTHING THAT WAS EVER ALIVE IN IT. We are also becoming a sedentary society that works hard all day long by sitting in front of a computer in an air-conditioned cubicle. I am not criticizing it, just stating the fact. And humans were never meant to do that. We evolved over those hundreds of thousands of years foraging and hunting. We were made to toil not sit around all day.

And our technological world has brought us plenty of other poisons too like bleach fumes, gasoline fumes, radioactive fallout from nuclear bomb tests and the reactor disasters of Chernobyl and Fukushima. And of course the destruction of the majority of the ozone layer by hair sprays. We sure do love to cobble up new chemicals and fancy machines and throw them around like there is no tomorrow. But there is a tomorrow and it always seems to bring us terrible news about the consequences of all of our fabulous creations.

The primary consequences of our actions are cancer and heart disease which are KILLING people by the hundreds of thousands each year. I would argue that many of those deaths are entirely PREVENTABLE too.

Right now one in three Americans will die of cancer, a disease that was one of the rarest known to medical science prior to World War II with only a handful – and I mean LESS THAN TEN – cases diagnosed by doctors each year. In the fifties these numbers exploded exponentially from hundreds per year to thousands to tens of thousands to hundreds of thousands of new cases each year. What changed? Two things: chemical additives to the foods we eat started appearing in the fifties and the nuclear bombs were set off in the mid forties through the fifties. These bombs create what we all know very well as the mushroom cloud, this thing sends radioactive fallout as high as 30 miles, that's the edge of space, and the upper atmospheric winds can distribute that fallout worldwide and it only takes ONE RADIOACTIVE ATOM to be absorbed by you, to ultimately possibly cause cancer in you.

Although we can't go back in time and stop all of the deadly radioactive contamination caused by the nuclear bomb tests and the catastrophic reactor failures, contamination that IS killing people with cancer worldwide and will continue to do so for thousands of years into the future, we CAN do something about the foods we eat and we can start exercising which plays a critical role in human health.

I continually harp about changing to a diet consisting of nothing but natural whole foods and there is a reason for that: these are the foods that we EVOLVED eating. Our species adapted to these foods over hundreds of thousands of years and our digestive tracts are literally made specifically to digest them and our bodies are made specifically to USE the vast array of molecules in them and they are NOT specifically designed to digest or use the constituents of TWINKIES, SODA POP or ROCKS (many minerals, if you have read Vol.3 – Minerals and Essential Nutrients, are provided as the oxides which are essentially rocks.) And we are still adapting to the SECONDARY FOODS that must be cooked in order to become edible in the case of plant foods and most dairy products which were added to our menu after we settled down and started farming and being able to feed livestock.

I am certain that almost every American who is not actively adding a solid well researched regimen of whole foods or supplements to their diet is MALNOURISHED. Three things are killing Americans:

1. They eat POISON in the form of CANCER CAUSING ADDITIVES to their PROCESSED foods on a DAILY BASIS. (And they are exposed to other POISONS also on a daily basis, like DIESEL ENGINE FUMES, HARSH CLEANER FUMES, etc.)
2. POOR DIET: even if you eat right, most of the plants are being grown in dead soil that has been overused for decades, the only reason the plants grow at all is because of the massive amounts of fertilizers being used on them – artificial, manufactured, chemical concoctions. This is what I affectionately call DIRTOPONICS. Just like HYDROPONICS or AEROPONICS, the plants must be given 100% of their nutritional requirements in order to grow, the only difference is that they are sitting in DEAD SOIL instead of pure water or air while they grow. Because of these conditions, many of the macro- and micro-minerals are dramatically reduced or completely missing, having been absorbed completely out of the soil by crops decades ago. Even the current crops, manage to eek out an existence based on their fertilizer sources of nutrients but cannot possibly be producing the supplements we expect from them in the quantities that they should have, hence we are all malnourished even if we eat the right foods because they simply no longer contain adequate, or natural, levels of the nutrients that they should be providing us.
3. LACK OF EXERCISE: You cannot expect to be healthy if all you do is sit in your car on the way to work. Sit at a desk all day at work, and sit at your TV all evening when you get home. You MUST find a way to do some aerobics, at least one hour DAILY.

This series is was originally meant to guide you through the bewildering maze of the vitamin shelf at your favorite drug store but I have since decided to expand on that greatly and try to not only answer all of the questions like "What is fiber and what is it good for?" but to also cover the many curative/preventative natural products out there and to provide simple, quick solutions to the basics of how to live a healthy happy and LONGER LIFE that is actually worth living.

These books are certainly not a substitute for professional advice. If you are currently on medication of any kind, you MUST CONSULT A DOCTOR before taking anything, including vitamins or any other supplements because they STRONGLY AFFECT the way your body works and can actually cause a VERY BAD REACTION in combination with certain strong medications.

Also, vitamins and minerals are ONLY THE BEGINNING; there are a multitude of ESSENTIAL NUTRIENTS that are neither vitamins nor minerals. Furthermore, MANY nutrients are NOT currently considered ESSENTIAL when they really ought to be and MOST of the phytonutrients that I cover in Vol.4 fall into this category. Eating right can prevent and heal just about any chronic malady including high cholesterol too.

This is probably the number one item that everyone is concerned about especially since the late 70's and early 80's when studies linked it with heart disease and heart failure. So now everybody lives in a hyped up panic about it and has their blood checked constantly for it and desperately avoids all of the sinister evil foods that contain it.

But what is it? I mean beyond the well known (now, but not back then when it was first announced that it was "deadly" as were eggs) "good" cholesterol and "bad" cholesterol. That still doesn't answer the question of what it actually is.

Time for a little chemistry. Anything that ends in "-ol" is by definition an ALCOHOL. So ethanol is ethane but converted into an alcohol which means that one of the hydrogen atoms attached to one of the carbon atoms was replaced by an oxygen atom with a hydrogen sticking out of it like this:

ALCOHOL MOLECULAR STRUCTURE

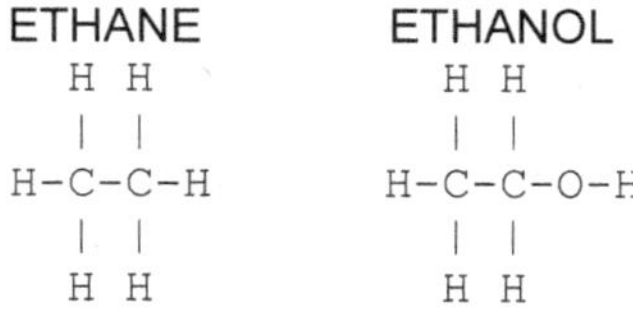

Ethane is a simple hydrocarbon containing only hydrogen and carbon, but ethanol, because the hydrogen atom was replaced by that –O-H group is a carbohydrate containing carbon, hydrogen and oxygen. So alcohols are carbohydrates, but they are also very polar in nature, that –O-H group gives them a positively charged end compared to the other end of the molecule which makes them excellent solvents and strongly chemically reactive compounds in general.

There are myriad naturally occurring alcohols in plants for example, geraniol, found in geraniums long ago before they hybridized it out of them or thymol found in thyme and one of the active ingredients in mouthwash (a powerful antiseptic.)

By now you should see where this is going; cholesterOL is an alcohol. However, it is a huge molecule and basically a form of fat (which are huge carbohydrate molecules, but it does have at least one –O-H group sticking out of it which is why it gets the –ol ending in its name.

So we know what it is, a fat molecule that is also an alcohol, but what does it do? Cholesterol is manufactured within the human body and it serves as the lubricant between the muscle fibers in every muscle in the human body. Even if you never ate a single molecule of cholesterol in your entire life, every muscle in your body would be bathed in cholesterol so that the muscle fibers could slide past each other easily rather than create friction and tear themselves to pieces.

Since plants don't have muscles it is a fair bet that they don't have much cholesterol in them and you would be quite right: they have absolutely ZERO. Cholesterol is an animal muscle tissue thing, so plants do not have any.

The key issue here is that we manufacture it ourselves and we make a lot of it and it is always present in the blood whether you eat nothing but plants or not. But if you do eat foods high in cholesterol, your body knows what it is – that it is a "good" molecule that it makes and it is not going to pass it up and it will absorb it from the foods you eat. Then it goes straight to the liver.

Now the story gets complicated. So you have all of the cholesterol that your body already makes in abundance, AND you have all of the cholesterol in the foods you just ate stacked up in the liver. The liver is NOT a storage warehouse, just a regulator valve. So over time it will release all of the cholesterol you ate into the bloodstream. Many tissues need it and they will pick it up, that's why it is always in the bloodstream whether you eat foods with it or not. But if there is an excess, more than what the various tissues need and therefore absorb, then this stuff can and will start to pile up in the bloodstream and also get packed away in the fat stores as they grow as well.

However, the cholesterol is not stored for the calories like the fat, it is just stored because is it useful and there is an excess of it. And this is an important consideration: obesity and high cholesterol are often related because of the person's diet and lifestyle, but the two are not directly related to each other at all. Skinny people can have high cholesterol and heavy people can have acceptable levels although both scenarios are relatively rare, they can and do occur because the two are not directly related to each other; fat and cholesterol serve two completely different functions in the human body. It is entirely because we already make it ourselves that eating a high cholesterol diet can lead to dire consequences.

We are also aware of the "good" and the "bad" cholesterols also known as LDL or Low Density Lipids, the "bad" ones, and HDL or High Density Lipids, the good ones. The actual terms are Low Density and High Density Lipoproteins. I just say "Lipids" because the term is clear and easy to remember: Lipid means FAT. We don't really have to chase the differences down here except to know that the RATIO of them is critical and can get knocked out of whack by a very poor diet over a very long period of time. And once this ratio gets messed up and stays that way for long periods of time, the body sort of gets used to this condition and tends to just let it stay that way, and that is why people who have changed their diets, still have high LDL versus HDL levels in the blood and are encouraged to start taking one of those prescription drugs to control it; many of which have already been pulled from the market because they are strong and they mess with your body's chemistry and many of these products have over long periods of usage KILLED the patient. Talk about the cure being worse than the problem!

And this is COMPLETELY UNNECESSARY. Eventually the body will get back to the levels it should have IF – and this is a BIG IF – you STOP EATING TRASH FOODS, begin to exercise (CRITICAL) and START getting proper and complete nutrition in your diet.

So why is the exercise critical? Do you remember what the cholesterol is used for in the body? Muscle lubricant. If you use those muscles, then the muscle lubricant gets used up, just like oil in your car and has to be replenished. This creates an actual NEED for the cholesterol which will LOWER the levels of it wandering about in the blood doing nothing and piling up over time.

If you are really serious about taking care of your own cholesterol levels without the use of those dangerous nuisance drugs, then you must be prepared to exercise – it is an integral part of the therapy and possibly the second most critical component of success in the strategy behind STOPPING the TRASH CALORIE foods.

And there is a strategy to this endeavor. If an enemy had occupied an allied country, and we asked our generals what to do, one might say: "I am going to take my troops across the border and drive them out." The next one might say: "I am going to bomb the supply lines and cut off their supplies and starve them out." And the third might say: "I am going to move the fleet into range and start shelling and attacking their rear bases of operations to harass their occupational forces." So as the leader which one would you choose to do? ALL OF THEM OF COURSE! This is war. We do not want to mess around and fight the enemy for the sake of fighting them, we want them DEFEATED and we want victory as quickly as possible so every weapon and every soldier we can throw at the enemy in order to quickly overwhelm them is the ultimate strategy and that is exactly what we are going to do to the cholesterol issue: we are going to use every weapon in the arsenal and we are going to use them all in as much quantity and quality as we can in order to overwhelm this enemy and defeat it.

Any time anyone asks a doctor: "How can I prevent cancer?" Answer: "Proper diet and exercise." Any time anyone asks a doctor: "How can I prevent diabetes?" Answer: "Proper diet and exercise." Any time anyone asks a doctor: "How can I prevent high cholesterol?" Answer: "Proper diet and exercise." Are you starting to get the idea? And most people hear this and they don't know what a proper diet is, and they seem to conveniently ignore that last part: the EXERCISE part of the equation, and the best diet in the world will not save you from anything if you don't get up and start working and sweating: it is MANDATORY for good health.

END OF CHAPTER QUIZ
1. Cholesterol is:
    A. An alcohol.
    B. A carbohydrate
    C. A form of fat.
    D. All of the above.
    Answer: D. Cholesterol is a large fat molecule with at least one –O-H group sticking out which makes it technically speaking an alcohol. Both fats and alcohols are carbohydrates. (They contain carbon, hydrogen and oxygen.)
2. Where does cholesterol come from?
    A. Only from the foods we eat.
    B. Some comes from the foods we eat.
    C. We make it ourselves in the body.
    D. Both B and C.
    Answer: D. Both B and C. Cholesterol is made by the human body and it can also be found in the foods we eat.
3. We would expect the foods highest in cholesterol to be:
    A. Secondary foods like grains and legumes
    B. Raw edible foods like spinach and apples
    C. Animal foods like beef and chicken
    D. Both A and C.
    Answer: C. Cholesterol is an animal thing, no plant makes it, no plant needs it, and no plants have any in them. (As a rule, but nature is vast and strange, I am sure there is one weird plant out there with some in it, but for the most part most plants have none.)
4. The major function of cholesterol is:
    A. Aids digestion by physically scrubbing the intestinal lining
    B. Provides additional calories
    C. Provides nutrients
    D. Provides lubrication to all muscle tissues in the body.
    Answer: D. This is the primary function of cholesterol.
5. The ONLY way to get the amounts and ratios of the "good" and the "bad" cholesterols back to healthy ones is to:
    A. Stop eating poor quality, high cholesterol foods
    B. Start eating low cholesterol, healthy foods
    C. Exercise daily
    D. All of the above
    Answer: D. You cannot control your cholesterol until you force your body to USE it. And it uses it for muscle lubrication. So the more you work hard and exercise, the more those cholesterol levels will return to normal healthy levels and ratios. Lack of exercise will keep those levels bad. And proper diet is a must to help control your cholesterol.

If you are already taking prescription cholesterol medication you will have to discuss all of the natural "treatments" that I am going to give you with your doctor. Even small changes in your diet and adding a daily exercise workout should be mentioned to your doctor because these are significant changes that will HELP your cholesterol levels return to their proper levels and ratios and you are already taking a powerful medication intended to do that artificially. Being aware of what you are doing, the doctor can anticipate rapid changes and monitor you more closely in order to be able to change your dosage as this happens. Always work with your doctor, most are not money-grubbing fiends and do want to see you improve and even defeat your affliction. And most will rejoice if you announce to them that you are going to stop eating a dozen eggs for breakfast and a pound package of bacon on the side and that you are going to start exercising too.

All joking aside, and the joke is on me, by the way, I used to swear I was "Gonna eat my bacon and eggs breakfast 'til the day I die," until I realized that the day I die was getting closer with every pound of bacon I was buying at the store. It gets closer anyway, no need to go chasing after it!

Before I go forward with the basic strategy it is important to realize what it means when the doctor says you have high cholesterol. We know that the blood test measures LDL's or the "bad" cholesterol, HDL's or the "good" cholesterol, but it also measures triglycerides, a form of blood sugar as well. Any one of these can be higher than what the medical industry considers "normal" or the ratios between them could be incorrect or most likely it is a combination of these: elevated levels and incorrect proportions of them with respect to each other.

Furthermore and of greater significance to this discussion it is important to realize that "having high cholesterol" is NOT in and of itself a disease or affliction; rather it is a SYMPTOM.

And it is of great importance to know what these elevated and incorrect ratios of these substances in the blood are a symptom of: it is critical to find out the CAUSE. Only when the cause can be identified and thus dealt with directly, can a true CURE be applied that leads to an END of the affliction.

Now there are certainly many afflictions of the human body, both diseases and chronic ailments for which there are no known cures at this time. But it is also important to know that medicine is a science and as such, science has a very specific way of doing things. They like to identify CAUSE and EFFECT relationships. Throw the ball at a certain angle and velocity, then apply the particle kinematics formula and predict where the ball will land to within the discrepancy caused by air resistance and it works every time. Medicine also wants to identify the cause of the problem and it also wants to verify the solution. So patient "A" gets malady "X" and they want to apply treatment "M" and see him cured. But they want ALL patients to be cured by "M" and when that becomes sporadic and unpredictable; some people are cured, some stay the same and some get worse, then the effectiveness of "M" becomes doubtful.

This causes many potentially effective treatments to be discarded by the medical industry and of far greater concern is the fact that many very effective treatments will never be properly tested because they are natural remedies and no one wants to spend hundreds of millions of dollars conducting the proper clinical trials and applying the proper statistical scientific methods to those results for something like carrots, which cannot be PATENTED and then SOLD to people in order to prevent loss of eyesight.

This means that there is a planet-wide pharmacopoeia of treatments growing wild out there and many of them are very likely the cures of just about every malady mankind suffers, and the pharmaceutical companies have people trudging through the Amazon Rain Forest in search of them, but not to give to you to cure you: but to ISOLATE the EFFECTIVE or ACTIVE compound within them and then chemically synthesize it from scratch in their Frankenstein labs. Only then could they SELL it. Otherwise it is of absolutely no interest to them because it would be of absolutely no VALUE to them. A further hindrance is the fact that many such wild treatments are severely diminished when they are isolated from the original plant which contains countless other molecules and those might be critical to the effectiveness of the active ingredient and without them, the results become unpredictable or the active ingredient becomes completely useless.

And even though we have made great strides in modern times concerning our ability to analyze a chemical compound and determine the atoms in it and their arrangement in the molecules, the fact remains that there are countless molecules in nature, in biology in particular, that still defy analysis. In fact we have only scratched the surface of molecular biochemistry. There are likely a thousand known compounds, in living things that we cannot yet analyze, for every one that we have analyzed so far.

And even if we could turn on a futuristic scanner that could map the molecule effortlessly every time, we still would not know how pairs of molecules present in any plant affect each other within our digestive tract or bloodstream. When we take those possibilities into account, then the possibilities explode exponentially from hundreds of compounds in the plant to trillions of possible COMBINATIONS in specific ratios that must be tested.

This is why I believe we will never know the ful extent of what is out there; we can know that something works, that it is an effective treatment, but we may never know WHY it is effective And this is a serious problem to us because it is a serious problem for the scientists and the profiteers. The scientists will refuse to ENDORSE the treatment and the profiteers will refuse to TEST it because they can't SELL it.

And this brings us back to the current discussion; we must first determine the CAUSE of the high cholesterol before we can proceed and since the LIVER is the one that makes the LDL's and the HDL's and the triglycerides and it is also the organ that releases into the bloodstream the contents of everything we eat then there are exactly four possibilities as to the cause of high cholesterol in the blood:

1) LIVER MALFUNCTION: The liver could be diseased, irritated or damaged in some way.
2) POOR DIET: The liver could simply be pushing a bunch of trash into the blood coming from the trash in the diet.
3) POOR HEALTH: Some other malady is affecting the levels.
4) A COMBINATION OF the first two problems: Chronic poor diet can indeed irritate the liver and cause it to malfunction as it dumps an endless supply of trash from the trash diet into the blood.

Knowing this and knowing that the vast majority of all processed and packaged foods are indeed trash foods that are terrible for your health and terrible for the liver, then it stands to reason that the EASIEST possibility to repair is number 2: POOR DIET. Although we cannot know for sure what specifically could be the trouble in number 3: POOR HEALTH, we do know that many people in modern times lead sedentary lifestyles which leads to poor cardiovascular health and that can and does affect these cholesterol levels. Poor health can also be caused by poor nutrition and the dietary changes I will be suggesting are certainly aimed at fixing those kinds of problems as well.

So the entire general strategy that was laid out in the preceding chapter is actually intended to address these two issues: poor diet and poor cardiovascular health because they are the easiest ones to repair on your own and now we will quickly recap and then get down to specifics:

1) STOP EATING packaged and processed foods – They are laced with cancer causing chemicals and processed forms of secondary foods like white flour which are nothing but TRASH CALORIES anyway and they do NOTHING GOOD for your health.

2) STOP EATING high cholesterol foods and we all know which ones they are: pork, eggs, beef, and chicken with the skin are at the top of the list, but virtually ALL animal meat has cholesterol in it including lamb (the top land animal food you can eat) and fish (the top form of animal meat.) I definitely do not recommend that you become a vegetarian, you still need COMPLETE PROTEIN (which contains all nine essential amino acids) and that is ONLY FOUND in animal meat. So, for the short

term – while trying to repair the high levels and poor ratios of the bad and the good cholesterols in your body, you will have to stick strictly to fish: it is the best kind of animal meat to eat anyway. If you can't do that, then very lean beef or skinned chicken are the second best choices.

3) START a high quality diet intended to help fight the high cholesterol. That is the subject of the upcoming chapters.

4) EXERCISE – I am certainly not a health and wellness major, all I can say is that if you want to exercise in the privacy of your own home like me, then you can buy those celebrity exercise tapes and hop around the living room (nothing wrong with that if it works for you) or get one of those exercise treadmills, rowing machines, or "exercycle" bicycles, and workout for at least one hour a day: GET IT DONE.

One last note concerning the exercise: I do not mean that you have to begin body-building and turn yourself into Arnold Schwarzeneggar even though most professionals do advise strength based workouts or what they call "burst" workouts. Building muscle mass will definitely lower cholesterol because you have more muscle tissue which means it must be drawn out of the blood and into that new muscle mass, but there is a limit as to how far that can go: will you continue to increase muscle mass until you become the size of a house? All I am talking about is simple aerobics. Just get yourself breathing heavily and sweating. Sweating is one of the ways the body detoxifies – its GOOD FOR YOU. The primary goal is to improve cardiovascular health because it can and does affect your cholesterol levels and if the increased muscular activity helps the body consume a little cholesterol along the way then that is a bonus.

If you have been very inactive for a very long time, then you should get one of those wrist heart monitors and ease into your exercise regimen: no sense in jumping on a treadmill and exercising yourself right into the emergency room on day one with a heart attack!

The trash calories interfere with the liver forcing it to temporaily warehouse large amounts of molecules and metabolize them all into forms fit for the bloodstream including glucose and the triglycerides. Because it is spending so much effort doing this it also interferes with the construction of new cholesterol molecules which it them has to package into molecular bundles: the LDL's and HDL's for release into the bloodstream and this is exactly why these foods loaded with processed sugars, high fructose corn syrup, starch and fats are terrible. Of even greater concern are the hydrogenated vegetable oils showing up in most packaged and processed foods which are ARTIFICIAL ANIMAL FAT. Natural animal fat is a waxy solid at room temperature, but plant fat or polyunsaturated fat is liquid at room temperature (vegetable oils) but people do not want to see saturated fat or pig lard in the ingredients in their foods, so the manucaturers put hydrogenated vegetable oil in them which sound nicer but it is still vegetable oil that has been artificially converted into a higher density fat that mimics animal fat and is solid at room temperature. However, the liver does not recognize these molecules and doesn't know how to metabolize them correctly which means they are TOXIC to the liver.

Rather than waste the time, money, energy, and space in your stomach on this garbage, let's start filling your digestive tract with foods that are going to help fix you up rather than help kill you, shall we?

1) ELIMINATE SECONDARY FOODS – Most of these are actually nothing but nature's TRASH CALORIES too including most grains, roots and beans – anything that must be cooked in order to become edible. The notable exceptions are old-fashioned oats, wheat germ, some of the dairy products and the legumes including green peas, chick peas and peanuts. But Rice, Corn, white wheat flour products, potatoes, and all beans are OFF THE TABLE for now.

2) START EATING raw edible natural whole foods including lettuce, cabbage, kale, collards, spinach, carrots, and most of the cucurbits (cucumbers, yellow squash, zucchini, and by the way watermelon and cantaloupe are in the family too!) Green beans are actually edible raw, they just don't taste very good, and I do prefer to cook my broccoli and cauliflower as well. Cooking these foods is fine, the point is that are all edible raw and the very best foods for you on Earth because of that.

In the meantime, we need to start working on those foods that are actually going to help reduce cholesterol and number one on the list is old-fashioned oats, NOT instant. I don't know what they did to the oats to make them instant and I really don't care either because the REAL oats only take about 10 minutes to cook up anyway. Even though there are many breakfast cereals that are actually very healthy choices, they are ALL OFF THE TABLE while we are at WAR: remember that we want to use EVERY WEAPON at our disposal in order to overwhelm the enemy and ensure a QUICK victory. So there is no time to mess around. You can get back to your favorite breakfast cereal AFTER the WAR is OVER.

FOODS THAT LOWER CHOLESTEROL

1) OATMEAL – So what is now for breakfast? Old-fashioned oatmeal. Why? Oats are high in fiber and fiber sticks to cholesterol and prevents its absorption in the intestines. Cholesterol is manufactured in the liver in the first place, not in the actual muscle tissues themselves. This is why it is always found in the bloodstream. The liver makes it and sends it out in the blood to the rest of the body. Keeping it out of our foods and therefore keeping it from ever reaching the liver in the first place will encourage the liver to get back to making it in the correct amounts and ratios. [2][3]

2) APPLES – Apples are high in fiber and antioxidants as well but only when eaten fresh and raw. You must eat WHITE apple flesh, never brown. Once the apple flesh has turned brown, some of the antioxidant powers have been LOST. Cooking anything reduces the fiber and thus reduces the ability of the food to absorb cholesterol in the intestines. (Old Ben Franklin had it right; an apple a day WILL keep the doctor away.)[2]

3) GARLIC – The sulfur compounds in garlic help to reduce the LDL cholesterol levels in the blood. Garlic is one of the top "heart" friendly foods on Earth because of this. While cooking with it is exquisite (as far as I am concerned) you should also take a garlic supplement as well. There is some concern about overdosing on garlic but 500mg or even 1000mg per day in addition to cooking with it is the way to go. Incidentally, sulfur compounds must also be regulated in the body and require molybdenum rich foods to help you do that: oats are rich in molybdenum. (This is a well thought out strategy, not just a "cut-and-paste" job.)[1][4]

4) ONIONS – The more the merrier, you can't overdose on these guys. I put them into every stew, boiled veggie and salad and they have the same powers as garlic: sulfur rich compounds that lower the "bad" cholesterol.[1]

5) WALNUTS – Just an 1 ounce per day brings over 2600mg of Alpha-Linoleic acid (ALA) a.k.a. the PLANT OMEGA-3. OMEGA-3 is a critical weapon in the war on cholesterol. Get walnuts preferably dry roasted, no salt, and shelled, and eat 1 oz of the kernels per day for a huge dose of this very cardiovascular friendly nutrition.[1][5]

6) FISH – About 4 to 5oz. per day. The preferred choice is Atlantic mackerel which will bring you 4,000 to 5,000mg of Omega-3 in the forms of EPA and DHA (the names are huge, and don't really matter.) These two are ONLY FOUND IN FISH and they are IMPORTANT to controlling cholesterol even though the fish have a lot of cholesterol in them – but so does every other form of meat and they DO NOT have any Omega-3 in them either. Furthermore, you must get COMPLETE PROTEIN daily as well because it contains the amino acid Threonine which has been linked to proper heart and liver health. Tuna, wild-caught salmon and cod as well as sardines are also good choices.[1][6][7]

The rest of your daily diet should consist of fresh tossed salads with only a touch of oil and vinegar dressing and the sides should have NO RICE and NO POTATOES. Boiled or preferably steamed veggies like yellow squash, cabbage, broccoli, spinach, cauliflower, etc. are a must. All of these have fiber, vitamins and other phytonutrients and are relatively low on TRASH CALORIES like starches and sugars. You don't need any more fat or oils in your foods either because the fish and the walnuts are bringing plenty of those. Oh, and put away the fry pan too. Even frying in an excellent oil like Canola (that and safflower are the ONLY ones you should ever use, by the way) and with no TRASH CALORIE breading (white flour or corn flour based) is still going to bring a lot of OMEGA-6's (that's what vegetable oils are loaded with) and the EFFECTIVENESS of the OMEGA-3's GOES DOWN if you are getting too many OMEGA-6's.

While we are stopping the eggs, don't forget that mayonnaise and salad dressing, as well as most dips and even pasta are made from eggs and the raw egg whites (in particular, yolks are not nearly as bad) in mayonnaise is TERRIBLE and must be stopped permanently. Trust me, I am having a real hard time shutting it down. They make something called "vegennaise" which apparently has no raw egg in it. I am hesitant to try it, because if like most vegetarian substitutes, it sucks, then I will always be drawn to mayonnaise. While you are trying to fix your cholesterol you must not eat ANYTHING made from eggs, period.

Still concerned that the Omega-3 (EPA and DHA) are not high enough? One tablespoon of Cod Liver Oil per day will fix that and make sure you get over 2600mg of it for the day. DO NOT OVERDO IT because CLO is loaded with straight up Vitamin A which you can overdose and it will be miserable and takes days to wear off. Take the single tablespoon per day especially if you are not going to eat fish for the day OR you just want to get as much of the best form (EPA and DHA) Omega-3's. Fish oil pills are OK , I even recommend them, but don't forget that getting those Omega-3's from the natural source is better. The fish have another constituent in their flesh that actually assists in the absorption of the Omega-3's and processed pills may be lacking in this trace constituent. ALWAYS EAT NATURAL WHOLE FOODS FIRST before considering any supplement no matter how good it is or how good it sounds. We were raised for millions of years on these foods and we depend on THEM, not processed packaged foods or refined pills to get ALL that we need.

END OF CHAPTER QUIZ
1. The one thing not in your diet that is critical to correcting bad cholesterol is:
    A. Getting plenty of sunlight each day
    B. Getting plenty of rest each night.
    C. Getting in an hour of aerobic exercise daily.
    D. All of the above.
    Answer: C. You must exercise in order to control your cholesterol and improve overall cardiovascular health. The sunlight helps you to produce Vitamin D3 and plenty of rest won't hurt either.
2. Which of the following foods should be avoided at all costs?

A. Trash calories like sugary snacks and starchy foods.
B. Mayonnaise and salad dressings and dips
C. Soda pop
D. All of the above

Answer: D. The trash calories are simply unnecessary and have been shown to worsen cholesterol levels anyway and this includes candy, cookies, cakes, pastries, rice, potatoes and so on. Mayo and its kin are made from raw eggs and they bind with the B vitamins and prevent their absorption which makes your cholesterol levels a LOT worse; avoid these like the plague. Soda messes with your stomach pH and therefore messes with your ability to digest and absorb everything you try to eat. Drop this nuisance forever and you will be far healthier for it.

3. Which of the following will help fight high cholesterol?
A. Foods high in fiber.
B. Foods high in the Omega-3 fatty acids
C. Foods high in sulfur.
D. All of the above

Answer: D. Oatmeal and fresh white pulp apples are excellent high fiber foods. Walnuts and most oily fish like mackerel, tuna, sardines, cod, etc. are all loaded with Omega-3 which helps lower cholesterol. Foods high in sulfur like garlic and onions as well as cabbage, cauliflower and broccoli, all help fight cholesterol although garlic is number one amongst them.

4. Fish are the only source of what essential nutrient (and we need a lot of it on a daily basis)?
A. Complete Protein
B. Iodine
C. Omega-3 (DHA and EPA)
D. All of the above

Answer: C. Although fish are the number one choice for a cholesterol reducing diet and they do contain Complete Protein, it is not the primary reason for eating them. Iodine is indeed necessary improving overall health and many fish do have traces of it, it is not the primary reason why you should only eat fish. The Omega-3 fatty acids DHA and EPA are only found in fish and we need a lot of them on a daily basis. The FDA is currently still attempting to establish an RDA for the Omega-3's and they are considering a number between 500mg and 1000mg per day and they are always conservative in their recommendations. The only plant source Omega-3 is called alpha-Linoleic acid or ALA and it is almost only found in certain nuts which most people do not eat on a daily basis either. This is exactly why most Americans are suffering from high cholesterol AND poor cardiovascular health; The Omega-3's help with both issues and are ESSENTIAL nutrients not OPTIONAL ones, and yet most people don't get ANY for

weeks, months and even YEARS at a time.
5. Having high cholesterol means:
    A. Having elevated amounts of LDL's in the blood
    B. Having elevated levels of either LDL's, HDL's or triglycerides in the blood.
    C. Having incorrect ratios of the LDL's, HDL's and/or triglycerides in the blood
    D. Both B and/or C
    Answer: D. Having high cholesterol can involve the elevated level of any one, two or all three of these blood constituents as well as incorrect ratios of them with respect to each other. Most people have elevated levels of all three and they are in the incorrect ratios. The correct ratio of LDL's to HDL's is actually 2:1. That means there are TWICE AS MANY "bad" LDL's in the blood as the "good" HDL's and that is considered "normal." However, when this ratio goes up, then it is really bad and having an excess of any of the three is definitely bad.
6. High cholesterol is:
    A. A disease
    B. A symptom of liver disease
    C. A symptom of poor diet and poor health
    D. Either B or C
    Answer: D. High cholesterol is a symptom, not a disease. It can be a symptom of serious problems with the liver or it can be the result of a chronic poor diet and poor health, especially poor cardiovascular health or poor health of other bodily systems caused by chronic poor nutrition from a poor diet.
7. The causes of high cholesterol that you can fix yourself are:
    A. Poor diet high in trash calories and cholesterol
    B. Poor diet with little essential nutrients needed to keep cholesterol in check
    C. Poor cardiovascular health
    D. All of the above
    Answer: D. You can change your diet and thus eliminate the trash calories and the high cholesterol foods and include a much more nutritious array of foods that can improve overall health and assist the body in maintaining proper cholesterol levels. And exercise will definitely improve cardiovascular health too.
8. All cholesterol in the blood comes from:
    A. The foods you eat
    B. The liver makes it
    C. Both A and B
    D. Neither A nor B
    Answer: C. The liver makes cholesterol and releases it into the blood stream but all of the cholesterol that you eat will also be released by the liver into the blood. This is why it is critical to cut it way down in your diet.

Since it is the liver that makes the cholesterol in the first place and the one that handles all of the cholesterol we absorb from the foods we eat, it makes sense that liver health should be a top priority.

1) NO ALCOHOL – This poison damages the liver and is the worst impediment to its proper health. If you really want to SAVE YOUR LIFE, then quit. If I can, anyone can and GOOD RIDDANCE to that mind-numbing DEPRESSANT anyway!

2) NO TRASH CALORIE FOODS – This places a huge burden on the liver having to sort through all of those garbage calories and store them up for later release and it also has to filter out all of those manmade artificial colors, flavors, preservatives and so on because it does not recognize them so it has to stop them all and most of them cause cancer and very likely KILL LIVER CELLS in the process.

3) B VITAMINS – While I strongly advocate getting ALL vitamins and minerals from the natural whole foods we eat, that would seriously increase your caloric intake and put the liver to work harder getting them out of those foods. Almost ALL Vitamin B Complex supplements contain CYANOCOBALAMIN which is a synthetic version of vitamin B12 and I strongly urge everyone against taking that junk. But you will need to take roughly 300% of the RDA (Recommended Daily Allowance) of Vitamin B3 – NIACIN at the very least. Niacin reduces the bad cholesterol in the bloodstream and therefore throughout the body by helping to convert it into the good one.

4) MILK THISTLE – This plant, a weed actually, contains SILYMARIN which is a known liver tonic that helps the liver detoxify and heal. Take the recommended amount on the bottle daily at first for a month or two, then back off to every other day, for a month or two and then back off to once or twice a week for proper liver maintenance.[8]

5) NO CAFFEINE – I will always have my morning cup of coffee, but that is a serious reduction from the way I used to suck it down all day long. You will have to make the same sacrifice. It is good for the liver to reduce caffeine as much as possible and coffee increases the levels of bad cholesterol and should be avoided.

STOP POISONING YOUR LIVER

There's no need to get into the details of the adverse effect of alcohol on the liver. It is a very well known fact that alcohol damages the liver and causes cirrhosis of the liver (extensive damage to the point at which the liver can no longer repair itself.) Alcohol is a terrible chronic poison to the human body and it completely upsets the liver and messes with all of its functions and since the manufacture of cholesterol is one of the big functions of the liver you can bet that drinking alcohol will mess with those critical blood cholesterol levels. It's got to go if you want to fix this issue and don't forget that those strong medications, for fixing the cholesterol, mess with the cholesterol levels which means they mess with the liver. Rather than try to force the liver to do the right thing while it is under siege from alcohol and a terrible diet, the best action is to stop putting it through the wringer at least until the cholesterol issue is resolved.

TRASH CALORIES – PROCESSED, PACKAGED FOODS

Those trash calorie foods are nothing but trouble. And there is a reason we are drawn to them. Throughout our deep dark evolutionary past, the number one objective all day every day of the hunter-gatherer tribes was to find food, especially calories. That is exactly why high calorie foods are so delicious and why we crave them because our survival depended on finding them and gobbling up as much of them as we could stomach and in nature the high calorie foods are the fruits (loaded with sugar) and fats found in nuts but mainly animals. The trash calorie junk food manufacturers load up their foods with both because they are delicious and they know that people who buy their products will easily become addicted to them. It is basically a legal form of drug dealing, but instead of dope, they are trash calorie pushers. It is incredibly hard to stop too. I know; I was there.

If you are addicted to these trash calorie junk foods, you cannot simply throw them all in the trash can where they belong and walk away. The addiction can really start to give you panic cravings once you do that. The best bet is to REPLACE the junk food with healthy food.

HEALTHY SNACKING

The goal here is not simply to replace trash calorie foods but to also get essential vitamins and minerals into your daily routine in their natural forms which are by far the best.

1) SUNFLOWER SEED KERNELS – ½ cup a day brings roughly 100% RDA of Vitamins B1, B5 and E. Vitamin E is going to be covered in a coming chapter, suffice it to say that you need it and it is rare in most foods other than seeds and nuts. So the walnuts also have some but the sunflower seed kernels ensure that you get plenty. Sunflower seed kernels also bring 100% of the RDA of phosphorus and selenium. Selenium is another essential nutrient that will play a big part of your effort to correct cholesterol levels and is very rarely found in most foods.[9]

2) CARROTS – You can never go wrong eating carrots. I snack on them throughout the day. Just 1 medium sized carrot brings about 200% of the RDA of Vitamin A in the form of beta-carotene. In this form it is also an antioxidant and the more antioxidants you take in throughout the day, the better, not just for cholesterol control but for overall improved health.[10]

3) CELERY – This is a superb snack for those trying to also reduce their caloric intake and lose weight. It takes more calories

to digest celery than you get back out of it, so every celery stick you eat provides net negative calories. I know that many in the scientific and medical industry are arguing that there is no such thing as "Net negative calorie" foods, but they have FAR LOWER calories than potato chips and zero saturated fat and zero cholesterol, so eat as may of these as possible – I will cover them in the whole anti-cholesterol strategy recap in the last chapter. Since you will also NEED IODINE, you can sprinkle IODIZED SALT on them as a surefire way to get that IODINE too.[11][16]
4) RAISINS – These are dense nutrition loaded with antioxidants, iron and chromium, you can't go wrong with raisins.
5) PUMPKIN SEEDS – These also play a critical role in providing hard to find minerals: ZINC and COPPER. Try to sneak in a few ounces a day at least.[12]
6) DARK CHOCOLATE – Every time I bring it up, everyone thinks I am crazy, but dark chocolate is one of the densest natural sources of Iron on Earth. I try to eat 4 oz. per day which brings 100% RDA of Iron AND Magnesium. It takes a pound of beef liver to provide that much iron. But I am not talking about candy. That chocolate is watered down with milk and has too much processed sugar added to it turning it into trash calorie nonsense. I mean "Baker's Chocolate" found in the baking isle of the grocery store. Read the ingredients which must list just one ingredient: Cacao (or "Chocolate.") Others list a litany of garbage and are basically FAKE chocolate and WORTHLESS. True dark chocolate is quite bitter so I dip it in honey. Honey is one of the most powerful curative/preventative foods you could ever eat. I add plenty to my morning oatmeal as the sweetener instead of trash calorie white sugar which I don't even have in the house any more.[13]

I imagine that those who are the most hard-core snackers like me have plenty of excellent choices in this list to choose from so you have no excuses, just try to make sure that you get enough of each one from that list to satisfy your body's needs as well as your cravings for those other terrible foods that they have replaced.

THE NATURAL LIVER REMEDY

The MILK THISTLE is strong medicine for your liver. If you do not drink heavily as you enter into this plan, then stopping should be easy and you will only need about one month of taking the milk thistle daily as recommended on the bottle. Then you can back off to every other day for a month and then twice a week thereafter. This plan is also based on the fact that you will also change your diet and drop all trash calorie foods and drinks. Remember it makes no sense to patch holes in the wall if you continue to shoot your gun at it. The SILYMARIN in the milk thistle will help the liver heal, but only if you stop damaging it and trash calorie junk foods laced with artificial chemical additives do great damage to the liver, and are well known causes of high cholesterol because of this, and all of those junk foods calories also put a burden on the liver and mess with your cholesterol levels as well.

FIXING THE CHOLESTEROL RATIOS WITH NIACIN

It is important to remember that the ratio of the LDL's to HDL's is just as important as the total amounts in the blood. This ratio is dependent mainly on a healthy liver. However, the big blast of Vitamin B3 – Niacin is also aimed at setting this right as well. Niacin is used by the liver to convert the bad LDL cholesterol into the good HDL cholesterol. And although niacin is present in most foods, it is only found in most of them in trace amounts that will not reach the 100% RDA of it. Two of the richest sources of niacin are tuna fish and peanuts. But you need to eat 10 oz. of tuna to get about 100% of the RDA or about ½ cup of peanuts (or peanut butter) to get that much. While this is not an issue for me, I don't normally eat this much of either one of these because they are both going to load you up on calories in these quantities. Not to mention the fact that this is one of the primary weapons in our war on cholesterol and we need to get a LOT of it so that it can help with converting the LDL into HDL which is critical in adjusting the ratio of them from bad to good. As a result I do recommend around 250% to 500% of the RDA of niacin daily.[1]

While niacin in these amounts is not necessarily dangerous (no B vitamin is considered toxic not even in huge quantities far beyond this amount) some people do get a reaction to taking a big dose of it all at once. It causes a slight rash and a tingling or prickling sensation in the skin and the effect is called the "Niacin flush."[14]

If you can find natural source Vitamin B supplements (rather than synthetic) and you can tell if it is because the manufacturer will mention it with great emphasis if it is derived from a natural source, then this is far better than a synthetic. However, if you can't get natural source niacin, then even the synthetic is better than nothing in this particular case because you must take it and you must take a lot of it. If you take 100% RDA amount in a single pill and it doesn't bother you (no niacin flush) then take one when you wake and have breakfast, then space at least two and preferably four more throughout the day and take them with either a meal of a substantial snack. If you do get the niacin flush it is not necessarily dangerous, but you might as well back off because it is simply a sign of excess that the body is not actually using, so taking it beyond the flush is just a waste of the product. Still, try to take 3 pills containing 20mg (100% RDA amount) each daily.[

TRIGLYCERIDES

The third component that doctor's monitor is called triglycerides. These are a high energy carbohydrate fuel made by the liver and launched into the blood for the entire body to use. Whenever a cell needs it; it is always available. This level will definitely improve if you stick to the removal of ALL trash calorie foods and drinks and stick to the natural whole foods I have outlined and this will work towards giving your liver a break from these horrible foods and the poisons they bring and of course no piece of the plan will work if you are drinking any form of alcohol. Alcohol, even triple X white lightning moonshine is LOADED with sugar – BAD for you – and alcohol which is poisonous to the liver – also BAD for you. As long as you can stay away from that menace at least until you have fixed your cholesterol levels, then there is a very good chance that you will succeed.[1]

END OF CHAPTER QUIZ

1. The best natural remedial for the liver is:
   A. Honey
   B. Milk thistle
   C. Sunflower seed kernels
   D. None of the above
   Answer: B. Milk thistle which contains SILYMARIN which is a natural curative for the liver.

2. The worst thing for the liver is:
   A. Processed and packaged foods
   B. Carrots
   C. Alcohol
   D. Both A and C
   Answer: D. Processed and packaged foods are loaded with TRASH CALORIES and ARTIFICIAL ADDITIVES which conspire to make the liver work harder and can damage it too. Alcohol is a POISON to the liver and should be avoided while trying to repair the liver and bring it back to optimum health which in conjunction with a low cholesterol diet will help fix your cholesterol levels.

3. One of the only ways to get 100% RDA of iron (essential to the liver and obviously the blood) from a natural food is:
   A. Beef liver
   B. Sunflower seed kernels
   C. Oatmeal
   D. Dark chocolate
   Answer: D. Dark chocolate. 4 oz. contain 100% RDA of iron as well as magnesium; another mineral that is hard to get in sufficient quantities from natural whole foods.

4. Which of the following snack foods is number one if you are also trying to lose weight?
   A. Carrots
   B. Celery
   C. Sunflower seed kernels
   D. Raisins
   Answer: B. Celery is a common inexpensive "Net negative calorie" food; each celery stalk you eat makes you lose weight, not gain it. The other three are also highly nutritious.

High cholesterol starts with the liver, but the trouble isn't over automatically even if we can straighten out the diet and get the liver back to optimum health. High cholesterol is almost always related to liver health and a poor diet high in trash calories and cholesterol, but like many systems in the body, there are MANY different moving parts involved and HYPOTHYROIDISM plays a role in high cholesterol too.

WHAT IS HYPOTHYROIDISM?

The basic definition is underactive thyroid. And the thyroid is a master gland that controls other glands in the body as well as the metabolism of the entire body. Underactive thyroid therefore can have a cascade effect on the other glands all of which participate in the entire body by producing hormones that the body needs, and because the thyroid regulates metabolism throughout the body, underactive thyroid leads to lowered metabolism which causes lethargy or feelings of being weak and having no energy. It also causes people to be much more susceptible to cold temperatures and because the metabolic rate has fallen off, the person stores excess calories that are not being burned to maintain body heat and therefore it causes a tendency for obesity.

While hypothyroidism can have many causes including disease, the number one cause is a lack of proper nutrition and the thyroid is one of the weirdest organs in the human body because it has some very strange requirements indeed. The thyroid needs three important essential nutrients two of which are rare minerals that are not found in most foods: IODINE and SELENIUM.

Aside from the fact that these two minerals are relatively scarce in the Earth's crust, they are exceedingly scarce in most foods, but our thyroid gland depends on them because it makes its hormones with them and those hormones are then sent out in the bloodstream intended to be received by all of the cells in the body, so even though the thyroid gland needs the iodine and the selenium to make those hormones, all of the cells in the body are the intended recipients of those hormones, so really – ALL CELLS in the body need those nutrients.

While we may not need a lot of these trace minerals like we do calcium or magnesium, we still need them and when they are missing not just for a day, but for decades at a time, this tends to lead directly to hypothyroidism which in turn leads to obesity and a general tendency for the person to want to be inactive.

The reduced metabolism over the course of many years leads to severe weakening of the cardiovascular system mainly due to inactivity. And poor circulation and inactivity can and will lead to high levels of cholesterol. This in turn starts to build up as arterial plaque in the arteries that can ultimately lead to heart attack or stroke.

The World Health Organization estimates that at least 50% of the world's population does not get enough iodine in their daily diet, which means half of all people on Earth are experiencing chronic deficiency of iodine and are therefore very likely suffering from hypothyroidism as well. And this problem is not exclusive to the poor nations of Earth either; it is just as prevalent in the U.S. and the other "First World" countries as anywhere else. And I believe that iodine and selenium deficiencies are the primary cause of hypothyroidism and the resultant obesity in these countries as well.

GETTING THE THYROID BACK ON TRACK

The third essential nutrient required by the thyroid is called phenylalanine, an amino acid found in most proteins and certainly available in abundance in all Complete Proteins which are in turn found in all animal meats including fish.[7] But even the vegetarians are likely getting ample supplies of this nutrient in plant protein rich foods like seeds and nuts. And the diet I described above requires you to eat fish as the entrée for either lunch or dinner and nothing else, just to make sure you get a good dose of Omega-3 in the forms DHA and EPA daily. The names are ghastly, but if you must know: docosahexaenoic acid and eicosapentaenoic acid. (I did warn you the names were ghastly.) [15] And those fish bring an ample supply of COMPLETE PROTEIN loaded with all nine essential amino acids including phenylalanine, so that one is covered easily.

However, iodine and selenium in particular are not so easy to get. Fish do contain some iodine, but most fish do not necessarily contain enough and it can vary quite a bit from one fish to the next – even in the same species. Therefore iodine is an issue that must be addressed and the selenium is very rare in natural foods though fish have a lot of it in them too by the way so that must be taken care of as well.

1) IODINE – The simplest way to make sure you are getting enough is to consume one teaspoon of IODIZED SALT or SEA SALT per day. I put half a teaspoon in the morning oatmeal and use a little here and there at lunch, dinner, or snacking on celery. You also need the sodium contrary to popular buzz. The sodium is involved in the connections between the nerve endings and the muscles. Most people have virtually eliminated salt from their diet which is a good thing except that now they get no iodine. If you have eliminated all of the trash calorie processed packaged junk foods and buy ONLY unsalted canned foods, and the rest of your diet is nothing but natural whole foods, as it should be, then now it is time to get that 1 teaspoon of iodized salt BACK into your daily diet. An alternative is 2 cups of organic yogurt per day. Try to eat at least one cup per day but two is better because this is one way to get 100% RDA of calcium which is essential for proper bone health and to prevent another epidemic scourge in our society:

osteoporosis. Those 2 cups of organic yogurt also bring 100% RDA of iodine, but it must be organic (from grass-fed cows.)[16]
2) SELENIUM – ½ cup of sunflower seed kernels daily will do the trick while providing you with 100% RDA of phosphorus (also necessary for healthy bones and teeth) and Vitamins B1 – THIAMINE, B5 – PANTOTHENIC ACID and Vitamin E – alpha-TOCOPHEROL. All of these play critical roles in the human body and Vitamin E is vital for a healthy cardiovascular system. An alternative source of selenium would be just 2 to 3 Brazil nuts per day: they have the highest concentration of SELENIUM of any food. While all nuts and seeds contain some selenium, we are not out to get some of it, we are out to get ENOUGH to make sure that the thyroid gland has all that it needs to function properly.[18]

Incidentally, you must not megadose on either of these trace minerals. To do so can also upset the thyroid gland. Too much of either iodine or selenium can also lead to UNDERactive thyroid as well as overactive thyroid. BOTH are trouble so try to stick as close to the 100% RDA values for both without going too far overboard.

END OF CHAPTER QUIZ
1. Complete protein (4 to 5 oz. such as fish) will provide what essential nutrient to the thyroid gland:
  A. Iron
  B. Phenylalanine
  C. Magnesium
  D. Selenium
  Answer: B. Phenylalanine is an essential amino acid found in all animal protein in sufficient quantities to satisfy the needs of the thyroid gland as well as the construction of new proteins throughout the body. Selenium is needed by the thyroid but it is not found in complete protein.
2. The most readily available source of iodine to the average American is:
  A. Organic Yogurt
  B. Seaweed like kelp
  C. Brazil nuts
  D. Salt
  Answer: D. Salt, but only the IODIZED products which were introduced in the 1920's specifically to shore up epidemic iodine deficiency in the American public and most other "First World" countries followed suit. Sea salt is also high in iodine.
3. Which of the following are the best sources of selenium?
  A. Salt or organic yogurt
  B. Dark chocolate or beef liver
  C. Sunflower seeds or Brazil nuts
  D. Oily fish like Atlantic mackerel or tuna

Answer: C. ½ cup of sunflower seed kernels or just two Brazil nuts can satisfy your 100% RDA of selenium.

4. Which is the best source of iodine?
   A. Salt or organic yogurt
   B. Dark chocolate or beef liver
   C. Sunflower seeds or Brazil nuts
   D. Oily fish like Atlantic mackerel or tuna
   Answer: A. IODIZED or SEA salt is the most readily available source of iodine for most people and just 1 teaspoon contains enough. It takes about 2 cups of organic yogurt to provide the daily requirement of iodine but this also provides 100% RDA of calcium and most other foods do not have enough calcium in them to be practical (other than cheese of course.)

5. Which is the only source of the Omega-3 fatty acids known as DHA and EPA?
   A. Salt or organic yogurt
   B. Dark chocolate or beef liver
   C. Sunflower seeds or Brazil nuts
   D. Oily fish like Atlantic mackerel or tuna
   Answer: D. All fish have these two omega-3 fatty acids in them but the highest concentrations are found n the oily fish notably Atlantic mackerel (#1) as well as wild-caught salmon, tuna, cod, and sardines. Herring, and anchovies are also loaded with it, but most commercially available anchovies are so heavily salted that they are not worth eating for the Omega-3's in them.

.6. The top plant and animal sources of iron are:
   A. Salt or organic yogurt
   B. Dark chocolate or beef liver
   C. Sunflower seeds or Brazil nuts
   D. Oily fish like Atlantic mackerel or tuna
   Answer: B. All animal meat has some iron in it, but we happen to need a huge amount of it in comparison to what is in most foods. We need nearly a pound of beef liver (higher iron content than the meat) to get enough and it is truly amazing that something like 100% pure cacao dark chocolate is so rich in iron that it only takes 4 oz. to satisfy our 100% RDA of this critical essential mineral..

7. Hypothyroidism is caused by chronic deficiency of:
   A. Iodine
   B. Selenium
   C. Complete protein
   D. All of the above
   Answer: D. A chronic deficiency of any one of these essential nutrients can and will lead to hypothyroidism which not only encourages inactivity and obesity it also leads to high cholesterol levels as well.

This is one of the most complicated systems in the human body. And the reason is because we rely on it heavily especially for brain function. If the level drops too low you pass out; too high and the body's systems start to malfunction including those triglycerides which in turn affect the cholesterol levels: everything is connected it would seem.

The main reason you must change your diet away from processed packaged foods loaded with trash calories is because these wreak havoc on the blood sugar system raising insulin levels as well as triglyceride levels and once these levels get out of whack, the cholesterol levels will rise as well.

By eliminating the trash calorie food and drink (that's soda pop and booze) you have gone a long way toward straightening this mess out. Still, the system can use some help.

1) CHROMIUM – This trace mineral assists insulin and helps to correct blood sugar levels and utilization. I imagine that most people do not get nearly enough in their daily diet and chronic deficiency can certainly lead to late onset diabetes as well as severe blood sugar imbalance. Three 8 oz cups of 100% Concord grape juice contains the 100% RDA of this critical mineral. I personally don't like the taste of this juice very much and so I cut it half and half with ALOE VERA juice. The Aloe vera juice tastes like dishwashing soap but the two together seem to form a tolerable mixture though it is still an acquired taste I am told. Nevertheless three tall glasses of this per day will take care of the chromium and also flood your digestive tract with ALOE which is one of the top remedial foods on planet Earth. It is very gentle and fixes a lot of chronic digestive maladies and there are a lot of anecdotal (unverified by clinical studies) reports that it can even defeat digestive tract cancers. In the meantime, it certainly does more good than harm and the Concord grape juice is one of only two natural sources of a trace substance that actually dissolves plaque build up in the arterial walls and makes them more flexible too. Since arterial plaque build up starts from too much cholesterol in the blood, you can see that the grape juice does reduce it and it reduces it SIGNIFICANTLY while promoting proper insulin levels and function. Drink it. By the way, one cup of broccoli provides about 88% of the RDA of CHROMIUM and 1 teaspoon of fresh minced garlic another 12%. Garlic is loaded with it which is why it is such a powerful agent for the cardiovascular system and an excellent remedial for blood sugar related issues.[19]

2) COMPLETE PROTEIN – This contains the essential amino acid LEUCINE which has been linked to proper insulin function as well. So the 4 to 5 oz. of fish you will be eating daily provides ample amounts of this critical component to the blood sugar regulatory system as well.[7]

3) MAGNESIUM – This is another mineral that most people do not
get nearly enough of even though it is found in most plant foods. In
fact the chlorophyll molecule is based on a magnesium atom so
whenever you look out at a sea of green plants like a forest just
think about all of that green which is chlorophyll which in turn is a
molecule based on magnesium. Obviously a healthy whole food
diet including the green leafy vegetables like spinach and kale will
be loaded with magnesium, but it is still not enough to satisfy our
rather high daily requirement of this critical mineral. In fact we
need over 20 TIMES as much of it on a daily basis as we do iron.
Since the 4 oz. of pure 100% cacao bitter dark chocolate contains
100% of the RDA of this mineral; that will do the trick. By the way,
it is involved in countless enzymes throughout the entire body and
has been linked to proper insulin utilization: that's why it is an
important component in the strategy: fix the blood sugar which in
turn helps to fix the high cholesterol.[20]
4) VITAMIN K – (menaquinone or phylloquinone) This essential
nutrient has been linked to the proper utilization of insulin
throughout the body as well. (I did say that this is a very
complicated system with many moving parts!) Just ½ cup of raw
fresh spinach has 500% of the RDA of this vitamin. Although
spinach is definitely the King of the Vitamin K superfoods, most
green leafy vegetables especially the dark green ones (lettuce and
cabbage are seedlings of enormous vines and do contain some
Vitamin K. but not much) like kale (richest source of Vitamin K),
mustard, collard, and turnip greens are also loaded up with
Vitamin K. I recommend some spinach in your lunch salad as the
very best way to make sure that you are getting plenty of Vitamin
K. Many people believe that lots of Vitamin K will cause internal
blood clotting but this is simply not true.[21] The number one
nutrient related cause of internal blood clotting that causes heart
attacks and strokes is much more likely to be severe chronic
Vitamin E deficiency. We will talk about that in the next chapter.
5) CINNAMON – Cinnamon has been directly linked to proper
blood sugar levels. And I have even seen supplements that
include both Cinnamon and Chromium, the idea being that this will
provide the plant which contains some powerful remedials for
shoring up the maintenance of proper blood sugar levels while
providing 100% RDA of chromium which most people don't get in
their daily diet which also facilitates the cells ability to use insulin.
While I have no quarrels with this product I am concerned about
the form of the mineral in them. These are usually manufactured
chemicals even if they are "organic" molecules. Many in the health
profession are calling into question whether these forms are
actually usable or "biologically active" forms of the mineral. This is
why I strongly advise everyone to try to get all of their essential
nutrients from natural whole foods the way we have always gotten
them for countless millennia. Since the human race didn't go

extinct, it appears that those foods brought us all that we need in forms that are biologically active and available for us to use. By the way, Cinnamon has about 200 TIMES the antioxidant power of raw carrots too![22]

Even though we have covered a lot of ground here, the story is still incomplete. In the next chapter we will focus on cardiovascular system health in general which includes more essential nutrients that participate in the process because we are talking about blood pressure, blood vessel maintenance and heart muscle health as well. So, maintaining optimal cardiovascular health, the system that moves all of that blood around, certainly works in concert with these essential nutrients which directly support the blood sugar regulatory system.

Incidentally, hypothyroidism caused by chronic deficiencies of the nutrients needed by the thyroid results in a dramatic reduction in the metabolism which also affects and is affected by blood sugar issues; the metabolism cannot return to normal if the blood sugar issues are not addressed and vice versa. So the strategy here – to lower cholesterol – has a vast array of interlinked subsystems in the human body that all affect each other and conspire to cause or be caused by cholesterol issues. Scrimping on any one of them can definitely throw the whole effort out of whack and fall short of the goal to return your blood cholesterol to optimum levels.

END OF CHAPTER QUIZ
1. The most critical mineral needed for proper insulin function is:
    A. Chromium
    B. Magnesium
    C. Iron
    D. None of the above
    Answer: A. Chromium. But magnesium also plays a critical role in proper insulin utilization as well.
2. Your best source of Chromium is:
    A. Spinach
    B. Complete protein
    C. Organic Yogurt
    D. 100% natural Concord grape juice
    Answer: D. The Concord grape juice is critical to the strategy, it not only provides all of your daily requirement of Chromium (3 cups/day and don't scrimp) it also contains a trace constituent that dissolves arterial plaque slowly and safely.
3. Another natural food that is a powerful remedial that helps regulate blood sugar levels is:
    A. Citrus fruits
    B. Salt
    C. Cinnamon
    D. Aloe vera

Answer: C. Cinnamon. Studies have shown that cinnamon does indeed help to regulate blood sugar and I have a heaping teaspoon in my morning oatmeal or 1000mg in supplement capsules otherwise and I can FEEL IT WORK.

4. True or False: Natural Vitamin K found in spinach and other green leafy vegetables is the most likely cause of internal blood clotting which can cause heart attacks and strokes.

Answer: FALSE. Chronic deficiency of Vitamin K will lead to internal blood clotting and severe chronic Vitamin E deficiency is the most likely culprit.

5. What is the best natural whole food source of Magnesium?
A. 100% Concord grape juice
B. 100% Pure Dark chocolate
C. Aloe Vera
D. Organic yogurt

Answer: B. 4 oz. of pure cacao bitter dark chocolate contains 100% RDA of BOTH iron and magnesium and is the easiest way to get your fill of both of these essential minerals.

6. Aside from Chromium and Magnesium what other essential nutrient is required for proper blood sugar regulation?
A. Leucine
B. alpha-Tocopherol
C. Phylloquinone
D. Both A and C

Answer: D. Leucine, an amino acid found in complete protein, and Vitamin K are both linked to proper blood sugar levels and utilization throughout the body.

7. Which of the following could be taken as a natural supplement to support blood sugar levels and utilization by the body?
A. 100% Natural Garlic
B. 100% Natural Cinnamon
C. Both A and B
D. Neither A nor B

Answer: C. While both are highly recommended in their raw natural forms, they are spices which most people eat infrequently and only in small amounts, high quality supplements of both are highly recommended in order to get sufficient amounts that can help the body fight cholesterol.

8. None of the above blood sugar regulatory efforts will work if:
A. The thyroid issues are not also repaired
B. The liver issues are not also addressed
C. You Fail to exercise
D. All of the above

Answer: D. All of these subsystems in the human body depend on each other and affect each other often in dramatic ways. It is very important to correct as much as possible and to stick with it; chronic deficiencies can take years to completely correct.

The heart and the arteries and veins are the highways that transport everything we are discussing including the cholesterols and triglycerides being produced and released by the liver as well as all of the nutrients, blood sugar (glucose) and insulin produced in the pancreas and the various hormones produced by the thyroid. It stands to reason that if this system is not operating at optimum efficiency then nothing else in the strategy is going to work very well either.

Ironically, all of the things that we have been discussing are intended primarily to improve the cholesterol levels which in turn will dramatically improve the cardiovascular system, but while the blood cholesterols in particular are still high, this is a major deterrent to bringing the cardiovascular system back to optimum performance. It is a conundrum.

Still, everything that you do to help your heart and cardiovascular network, will have positive results even if it takes some time for the improvement to even become measurable. Many people balk at the notion that this strategy could take years before everything gets back to optimum health and ideal levels of the cholesterols and the triglycerides across the board. But this does not mean that the challenge is not worth the attempt or the wait: on the contrary, bringing your whole body and all of its systems back to ideal performance especially through a completely natural whole foods based diet and easy daily aerobic workout will pay tremendous dividends down the road because: 1) It keeps you off of those harsh "statin" drugs many of which have been discontinued because they KILLED the patients, 2) All of your bodily systems will be in far better health which tends to make you feel much better, get sick less often, and can help the body ward off cancer as well, 3) Being healthy and feeling healthy leads to greater happiness and contentment, 4) Being happier will pay off very well in the long run because you will get a longer run in this life due to your greatly improved health. Living longer, healthier and happier sounds like a pay off that is very well worth the effort and the wait to me.

ALL YOU NEED FOR THE CARDIOVASCULAR SYSTEM
1) ONE HOUR OF AEROBIC EXERCISE DAILY: That hour (minimum) of aerobics daily is a MUST. Personally, I despise exercise, especially when I was a landscaper and used to carry a gas powered weedeater around for seven hours during the day. If you have a job that actually gives you a decent workout like that (not sitting on a riding mower, but carrying the heavy tool all day while you work with it) then you might very well be getting all of the exercise you need on those work days, but do not scrimp on your days off.

2) CALCIUM – We know that calcium is used in the construction and maintenance of the bones and teeth, but did you know that it is also used in many other systems in the body and t is an integral construction material used in the arteries and veins as well? Arteries and veins are not actually alive in the sense that they are not made out of living cells like all of the other tissues in the body. They are made out of proteins and calcium based molecules that add strength to the walls. But they are not made out of tempered steel, so they do erode and need regular maintenance not only so they won't wear down to the point of having holes in them but also because they are plastic in nature as well and must remain both flexible (able to bend,) and malleable (able to stretch.) Anyone suffering from chronic calcium deficiency could suffer from bone loss and eventually such maladies as osteoporosis, not just because the bones need the calcium per se, but because they act as calcium repositories and will release calcium into the blood stream for use by other systems as needed including the continual maintenance on the arteries and veins themselves. Just because a person has stopped growing does not mean that the bones are complete and there is no longer any need for calcium; on the contrary they will wither over time as the bones give up their stores of calcium to the other systems that need it and that's the most likely cause of bone loss and osteoporosis. One cup of whole milk contains about 31% of the RDA of calcium. Personally I do not want to drink a quart of milk per day to get enough even though the milk is bringing it in an excellent natural form. The next best all natural whole food that brings calcium is cheese, preferably unprocessed and 3 to 5 ounces depending on the type will bring 100% of the RDA for calcium because we happen to need a LOT of calcium on a daily basis for ideal performance of all bodily systems that depend on it (Even the brain uses trace amounts of it.) I never recommend supplements because they are usually in the form of calcium phosphate (basically concrete cr bone, both are similar at the basic raw material level) and while we can get some of the calcium and the phosphorus out of this, even dogs have trouble digesting crunched up bones and their digestive tracts are optimized to deal with it (they are scavengers so their deep dark evolutionary past was spent gnawing on what the lions left for them: skeletons with bits and pieces still attached to the bones.) If you must rely on a supplement, Calcium citrate, calcium in an organic molecule, albeit manufactured, is the best way to go and certainly far better than calcium phosphate or worse calcium carbonate (limestone, by the way.)[23]

3) VITAMIN D3 – (cholecalciferol) If you are going to get all of the calcium that your body needs, you better make sure that you get enough Vitamin D3 as well. This vitamin is critical in that it assists the body in actually using all of that calcium. If you are short on Vitamin D3, then the calcium will still get absorbed, but the body will not be able to use it properly and that can lead to it building up in the arteries and veins and this can indeed contribute to arteriosclerosis (hardening of the arteries.) If you do not get enough calcium you will also get hardening of the arteries, because the calcium is used to keep them properly repaired and this maintenance is a continual and ongoing process throughout your lifetime. It is chronic Vitamin D3 deficiency that causes all of the trouble with our ability to properly USE the calcium we get in our diet that is leading to such maladies as arteriosclerosis and osteoporosis. Two 20 minute exposures to the sun with only your face and arms exposed should provide you with roughly 100% RDA of Vitamin D3. You cannot use sunblock though, because it is the ultraviolet rays that are needed to make the vitamin in the skin. We can make all we need because it is rather hard to find in sufficient quantities in natural foods other than dairy products which are highly processed secondary foods that I normally do not recommend other than organic yogurt and cheese. The same cup of whole milk does contain 31% of the RDA of natural vitamin D3 as well. The calcium and the vitamin D3 are at matching amounts because the baby cows have almost the same exact biochemistry for handling the calcium that humans do. If you are taking the tablespoon of Cod Liver Oil to bolster your Omega-3 DHA and EPA intake for the day which I highly recommend whether you are sticking to fish as your only source of complete protein or not, then that has 150% RDA of natural Vitamin D3 in it and you are good to go. Do NOT take any other form of the vitamin. We make D3 in our skin and that's the only form you should take (and it is the one in dairy and the Cod Liver Oil too.)[24][25]

4) MAGNESIUM – This has already been covered and getting your fill is a definite requirement for overall health but magnesium plays a role in the proper utilization of calcium as well. 4 oz. of 100% pure cacao bitter dark chocolate contains 100% RDA of this mineral which is difficult to get in the large amounts that the human body requires on a daily basis. It is #6 by weight needed daily or about 400mg which is over 20 TIMES more than our daily requirement of iron which we also have trouble getting in sufficient amounts.[20]

5) VITAMIN K – (phylloquinone or menaquinone) This is another essential nutrient already discussed and it plays a critical role in the blood and also assists in the utilization of calcium. ½ cup of raw spinach yields 500% of the RDA, but most other dark leafy greens like kale, mustard greens and turnip greens are loaded with it as well.[21]

6) LYSINE – This is another one of the nine essential amino acids found in sufficient quantities in 4 to 5 oz. of **Complete Protein** that is found in virtually all animal meats including the fish which is already on the menu. Lysine, however, is not so prevalent in plant proteins and vegetarians should be aware that they will need significantly more plant protein to make sure they are getting enough lysine and methionine (another essential amino acid that is not nearly as abundant in plant protein as it is in animal protein.) Lysine has been linked to the body's ability to properly use calcium as well.[7]

7) VITAMIN E – (alpha- or gamma-Tocopherol) One of the significant roles of vitamin E is that it prevents internal blood clotting which leads to atherosclerosis (plaque buid up in the arteries,) heart attacks and strokes. And I am certain that the majority of Americans have diets that are very low in Vitamin E and chronic deficiency can lead to any of these nasty consequences. Personally, I want no part of the dire results of chronic deficiency of this critical vitamin and it is almost exclusively found in seeds and nuts and nowhere else. The ½ cup of sunflower seeds has nearly the 100% RDA of this critical nutrient for your cardiovascular health. And chronic deficiency of Vitamin E is the far more likely culprit of heart attacks and strokes than overdosing on Vitamin K since most people don't even like spinach or mustard, collard, and turnip greens and likely get very little Vitamin K in their diets. Both of these vitamins (E and K) are required for proper nutritional support of an optimal cardiovascular system.[26]

8) COENZYME Q10 – (CoQ10) This is another health industry buzz word of late and it has been directly linked to heart health. We do make it ourselves and I am always hesitant of taking massive quantities of something that our own body's make because the body can become dependent on the supplement. In the case of all of the minerals, no living organism on Earth can manufacture them, that would require a nuclear process so only nuclear breeder reactors and stars can transform one kind of atom into another, so we do need to get all of our minerals from external sources whether they are natural whole foods or pills, but for organic molecules that we do manufacture ourselves like Vitamin D3, I always encourage people to let their bodies do the work and make it since they can. However, if you have spent a long time on a poor diet consisting of processed and packaged foods bringing far too many trash calories and artificial chemical additives, and have spent a long time relatively inactive, then you might want to take the CoQ10 at the recommended dosage on the bottle for a few months and taper off. I do recommend that you do this and I am aware that CoQ10 is very likely the most expensive item in the entire list of recommendations in this book; don't scrimp, your heart needs the boost as you transform your diet and lifestyle.[1]

9) THE OMEGA-3 FATTY ACIDS (DHA, EPA and ALA) The health industry is definitely in the midst of a total craze about these and for good reason too; the vast majority of Americans in particular are chronically deficient of these critical ESSENTIAL nutrients because we are beef eaters, not fish eaters. And NO

LAND ANIMAL provides ANY OMEGA-3. If the food product has it in it, then it has been added because the only animals on Earth that have Omega-3 DHA and EPA in them are the fish. All fish have both of these Omega-3's but the oily fish are LOADED with it and it is a critical component of repairing and maintaining your heart and cardiovascular health. It comes as no surprise to any health professional that the Japanese are, as a society, far healthier than any other society on Earth and the reason for that is their diet which consists primarily of PRIMARY plant foods (raw edible plants) and fish where they are getting a regular large dose of these healthy Omega-3's. 4 to 5 oz. of Atlantic mackerel, tuna, cod, wild-caught salmon or sardines per day plus 1 tablespoon of Cod Liver oil will make sure that you are getting a megadose of this very safe cardiovascular friendly pair of nutrients.

ALA or alpha-Linoleic acid, is also an Omega-3 fatty acid and it is the only one that can be found in foods other than fish and it is only found in certain seeds and nuts. The human body can convert ALA into DHA and EPA but it remains to be seen if the body can convert enough even if it is in ample supply in the diet, to adequately cover the body's needs for them. Nevertheless, we should also get our fill of ALA as well as DHA and EPA because the research into these nutrients is currently still under way and the FDA has yet to even make a determination as to what the RDA for the Omega-3's should be. 1 oz of walnuts per day will give you a big blast of about 2,600mg of this all important heart and cardiovascular friendly nutrient.[15]

10) POTASSIUM – This is very likely the number one mineral that most people on Earth are not getting enough of on a daily basis over the majority of their lives because we need a LOT of it. In fact, potassium has the largest RDA by weight of any essential nutrient other than water, air, useful calories to burn, and protein. The FDA's RDA for potassium is 3200mg, that's 3.2 grams or roughly a teaspoon of potassium chloride would be necessary to fulfill that requirement on a daily basis. And don't think that bananas, which everybody knows are high in potassium, will take care of the problem. One large banana contains approximately 14% of the RDA of potassium and it is one of the densest sources of this critical mineral. I am not going to eat SEVEN to EIGHT large bananas per day trying to fulfill my 100% RDA of potassium. But there is a way to get all of that potassium in a reasonable serving size on a daily basis: Low Sodium Vegetable Juice. They use potassium salt rather than sodium salt to maintain the desired salty flavor of the drink and it takes a lot more of it to compensate for the missing sodium salt. About 32 oz. of Low Sodium V-8 brand vegetable juice will cover your daily needs for potassium and it is CRITICAL. Potassium (and sodium, by the way) are involved in the synapses between the nerve endings and the muscle fibers and severe chronic deficiency can lead to acute potassium deficiency which manifests itself in uncontrollable muscle twitching (I used to get this a lot in my little finger and eyelids) as well as long powerful and unstoppable bouts of hiccups. This comes from malfunctions in those nerve endings so the nerves can no longer control the muscles and they start contracting out of control. Something that you NEVER WANT TO HAPPEN to the one muscle that keeps you alive: YOUR HEART. Your body will rob any and all other nerve-muscle connections for the potassium it needs to keep your heart beating properly, but it makes no sense to play with this issue. Oh and by the way, your daily exercise will mean that your body will have a higher demand of potassium than ever before and potassium doesn't just keep your heart beating properly either, potassium has been linked to maintaining proper blood pressure levels as well. And since almost everyone on Earth is not getting the huge amounts of potassium they need on a daily basis, this chronic deficiency, I believe, is the number one cause of heart attacks, heart disease and high blood pressure in the United States and indeed the rest of the world causing hundreds of thousands of EASILY PREVENTABLE DEATHS every year. So, get that Low Sodium V-8 (or whatever brand you prefer) read the serving size and amount it provides and make sure you get at least 100% RDA of potassium daily for the rest of your life. It will be a much longer healthier and happier life if you do.[27][28]

11) VINEGAR – Small amounts of vinegar have been shown to be highly effective at lowering blood pressure and while I will provide a litany of warnings at the end of the book it is VERY IMPORTANT that you DO NOT MESS WITH VINEGAR IF YOU ARE ON BLOOD PRESSURE MEDICATION. That harsh medication is already working to lower your blood pressure, adding vinegar which is the body's natural method of buffering the blood pH and of lowering the blood pressure as well could cause you to pass out from lowering it too far. With that said, people who do not drink alcohol and are not on blood pressure medication are ideal candidates for taking vinegar. White vinegar will work, it just tastes incredibly awful and most people choose apple cider vinegar which tastes just about as bad. Instead try red wine vinegar which is next to the olive oil in the supermarket. It too has a rather strong taste but it is both sweet and sour and I put a dab in my 100% Concord grape juice and also use it to make my own salad dressing. It doesn't take a lot, 1 tablespoon a day, and it is very effective.[29]

12) IRON – The World Health Organization estimates that 80% of the Earth's population is chronically deficient of this important mineral. Even the American beef eaters are not getting enough. Sure it is in the beef, but not enough to get you the 100% RDA requirement. Even Beef liver which is one of the densest sources of iron from any animal food would still take nearly a pound of it to get you that much iron. Many supplements that I checked a few years back contained iron in the form of "ferrous oxide" which I suppose is a politically correct way of saying RUST. Nowadays, the supplement manufacturers have apparently already been called out on this because it is basically useless (we can't digest RUST and only get about 1% of the iron that is in it) and now they are including it in such compounds as iron fumarate which is still manufactured, but at least it is an organic molecule. However, there are many health professionals that are still calling into question whether or not these manufactured organic molecules are providing the minerals in both a usable as well as a safe form. Because we can actually absorb pure iron in our digestive tract, I suspect that these organic molecules are providing it in a usable and safe form. However, the very best sources are still all-natural whole foods and the only three choices (in reasonable amounts) are clams, spirulina and 100% pure cacao bitter dark chocolate.

Just 3 oz. of spirulina will provide you with 100% RDA of iron, but it is blue-green algae and… ahem, it tastes like it too. 4 oz. of pure 100% cacao bitter dark chocolate (you can find it in the baking isle of the grocery store in "Baker's Chocolate" bars) is far more readily available to most consumers and I doubt there is a kid on the planet who would complain about having to eat it! However, pure cacao dark chocolate is very bitter so I dip it in all-natural bee honey. Although the honey is going to bring some calories, it is one of the most powerful curative/preventative foods on Earth, loaded with antifungal and antibacterial compounds that the body absorbs into the bloodstream that work wonders on helping the immune system and also with detoxification. I am constantly trying to invent excuses to eat more honey and it doesn't seem to bother our digestive tract bacteria at all either. Clams are the richest source of iron. Just 2.5 oz, will bring you 100% RDA of Iron. Canned clams are usually wild "caught" and perfect.[13][30][31]

Of course, I raise the issue of iron here because it is needed in order to make new blood cells and we are talking about cardiovascular health and these guys are the number one thing that the bloodstream was originally intended to transport. But iron is also in every muscle cell in the body as well in the form myoglobin. When the hemoglobin picks up an oxygen atom in the lungs it then transports it out to a capillary and that is where the myoglobin in the muscle cells can take the oxygen atom away from the hemoglobin molecule and store it until it is needed by the muscle cell to use it to burn a sugar molecule. So we don't just need the iron for the blood cells, we also need it for the muscle cells too, including the one muscle that we need to keep functioning every second of our lives: the HEART.[32]

13) SODIUM – Together with potassium, sodium is needed in the synapses between the nerve ending and the muscle cell and helps move the electron (the nerve signal) across to the muscle cell in order to control it. Normally sodium in the form of salt is overly abundant in the average American diet found everywhere from processed packaged foods and canned foods to restaurant foods. If you are changing your diet properly away from this kind of a diet to one consisting of only natural whole foods and "No salt" canned foods, then it is time to get some salt BACK into your diet. I have already recommended 1 teaspoon of IODIZED or SEA salt as the easiest way to make sure that you are getting enough IODINE for your thyroid gland to use. The amount is actually based on making sure you get enough SODIUM as well because all the potassium in the world will not help you if you do not get 2900mg of sodium per day (100% RDA) along with it. Those 2.9 grams are the second largest weight of any essential nutrient behind potassium so both are needed in huge amounts compared to most other nutrients. To give you an idea, you only need 18mg of iron daily. That means you need over 160 TIMES as much sodium on a daily basis.[27]

THE REST OF THE ESSENTIAL NUTRIENTS

Whew! That was a big list, but it is not over yet. Almost every single essential nutrient the body needs, is needed for a wide range of tasks and almost always crosses paths with another one such that if you are short on one, this has a domino effect causing you to be short on another one which it facilitates in some way like Vitamin D3 which is needed to coordinate the usage of calcium. It has also been found that Vitamin C assists in the absorption and utilization of most of the B vitamins. While we KNOW many of these interdependencies, many more are being investigated and discovered all the time. And there are very likely many other interdependencies between the known essential nutrients and others that are not considered essential like the many phytonutrients ranging from the carotenoids to the flavonoids which is why I strongly urge everyone to get their nutrients from all-natural whole food sources that contain all of these trace constituents in the exact proper amounts that can do their jobs ranging from helping us to absorb the nutrient in the digestive tract to helping them actually function in the bloodstream and even within the individual cells in the body.

But because of all of this interdependency, there is no way that we could ever leave out the remaining essential nutrients that I have not already listed, so you also need your 100% RDA's of Vitamin A, and C as well as phosphorus, manganese, zinc, copper, and chlorine although this last one is in the salt so it is already covered.

END OF CHAPTER QUIZ

1. The cardiovascular system is involved in high cholesterol in what way?

    A. It makes the bad cholesterol

B. It transports the cholesterol and can get damaged by excesses
C. Both A and B
D. Neither A nor B
Answer: B. The cholesterols are made in the liver. The cardiovascular system, including the heart and the arteries and veins, transports it to the muscles for use, but too much can and will damage it.

2. A common form of damage caused by excess cholesterol in the cardiovascular system is:
A. Atherosclerosis
B. Heart palpitations (irregular heart beat)
C. Osteoporosis
D. All of the above
Answer: A. Atherosclerosis or plaque build-up in the arteries is a direct result of excesses of cholesterol in the bloodstream. Arteriosclerosis or hardening of the arteries is caused by Calcium deficiency or deficiency of its many helpers.

3. Chronic deficiency or excess of this nutrient can cause arteriosclerosis:
A. Iron
B. Potassium
C. Sodium
D. Calcium
Answer: D. Calcium, Calcium is used to maintain the arterial walls throughout life. Shortages will prevent the proper structural maintenance of the blood vessel walls making them lose their elasticity and thus harden.

4. Chronic deficiency of Calcium can lead to:
A. Arteriosclerosis
B. Heart palpitations (irregular heart beat)
C. Osteoporosis
D. All of the above
Answer: C. Osteoporosis can be caused by chronic deficiency of Calcium especially for those who avoid dairy products which are the only calcium rich foods in our diet.

5. Which of the following plays an important role in our ability to properly utilize Calcium?
A. Magnesium
B. Vitamin D3
C. Vitamin K
D. All of the above
Answer: D. All of the above contribute to our ability to use the calcium we get in our foods. Shortages of any one of them can lead to a number of problems including arteriosclerosis or osteoporosis.

6. The #1 thing for improving your cardiovascular health is:
A. Aerobic Exercise

B. Elimination of poor foods in your diet
C. Proper nutritious diet
D. All of the above
Answer: A. Exercise. But eliminating foods high in trash calories laced with carcinogenic chemicals ard starting an all natural whole foods diet are just as important.

7. Which essential amino acid found in complete animal protein assists in the utilization of Calcium?
A. Methionine
B. Leucine
C. Phenylalanine
D. Lysine
Answer: D. Lysine found in sufficient quantities for the body in 4 to 5 oz. of any animal meat is a critical part of making sure that the calcium is properly put to work in the body.

8. Chronic deficiency of this nutrient is likely very high and can lead to cancer, heart attack and stroke.
A. Vitamin D3
B. Vitamin E
C. Vitamin K
D. Vitamin C
Answer: B. Proper amounts of Vitamin E assist the metabolism (a.k.a. the "Energy vitamin") and help prevent damage to DNA (shortages are likely one of the major causes of cancer) and prevent internal blood clotting which is why it can help prevent heart attacks and strokes.

9. The reason chronic Vitamin E deficiency is likely very high in the U. S. is because it is only found in significant quantities in:
A. Fish
B. Dark green leafy vegetables like spinach
C. Grapes, raisins and grape juice
D. Seeds and nuts
Answer: D. Most seeds and nuts have a lot of vitamin E and a few of them like sunflower seeds are loaded with it.

10. Coenzyme Q10 has been directly linked to:
A. The heart
B. The capillaries
C. The bones
D. The liver
Answer: A. CoQ10 has been directly linked to heart health.

11. Potassium is needed for:
A. Maintaining proper (lower) blood pressure
B. Maintaining proper heart muscle regulation
C. The synapses between the nerve endings and the muscle cells
D. All of the above
Answer: D. Potassium plays a critical role by serving as the electron mover in the synapses between the nerve endings

and the muscle cells. An acute deficiency can have life threatening consequences because the heart muscles will no longer be under control. Potassium has also been shown to play a significant role in lowering blood pressure as well.

12. The Omega-3's play a significant role in lowering cholesterol but can only be found in what food?
   A. Oatmeal
   B. Dark leafy vegetables like spinach
   C. Grapes, raisins, and grape juice
   D. Seeds and Nuts
   Answer: D. Some seeds and nuts are loaded with alpha-Linoleic acid (ALA) which is one of the Omega'3's. Just 1 oz of Walnuts has about 2600mg of ALA and is one of the few plant superfoods loaded with it.

13. The only food on Earth with Omega-3 DHA and EPA in it is:
   A. Fish
   B. Dark green leafy vegetables like spinach
   C. Grapes, raisins and grape juice
   D. Seeds and nuts
   Answer: A. All fish are the only source of DHA and EPA Omega-3 fatty acids although the oily fish: Atlantic mackerel, wild-caught salmon, tuna, cod and sardines are loaded with it.

14. Which of the following have been shown to help lower blood pressure?
   A. Sodium
   B. Potassium
   C. Vinegar
   D. Both B and C
   Answer: D. Proper levels of potassium and a little vinegar have both been shown to reduce high blood pressure.

15. We need large amounts of sodium on a daily basis and it plays a key role in conjunction with:
   A. Chromium
   B. Magnesium'
   C. Potassium
   D. We do not need sodium
   Answer: C, Both sodium and potassium form the "sodium-potassium pump" in the synapses between the nerve endings and the muscle cells which allows the brain to control them.

16. Which is #6 by weight amongst all daily essential nutrient requirements and is difficult to get in sufficient quantities daily?
   A. Iron
   B. Zinc
   C. Vitamin K
   D. Magnesium
   Answer: D. Magnesium. We need over 20 TIMES more magnesium every day than we do iron and it plays countless roles in cellular processes throughout the human body.

There are still more natural foods and extracts that have been shown to be effective at lowering cholesterol. Some of these work directly on the issue by serving as liver tonics (things that help the liver) while others get involved in more indirect pathways, and some are still under investigation to find out why they work at all. And that might be important to the scientists and the profiteers, but for now, we are only interested in things that work, even if the pathway they use is still a mystery.

FOODS and OTHER NATURAL PRODUCTS THAT HELP LOWER CHOLESTEROL

1) RED YEAST RICE – 1200mg twice per day has been shown to lower cholesterol by as much as 32%. This supplement comes highly recommended although I have never personally tried it but it could work wonders for you in conjunction with the natural whole food strategy I will lay out in the next chapter. Many RYR products have come under close scrutiny by the FDA recently because they contain a measurable amount of a regulated prescription statin drug. It is likely naturally produced by the red yeast and also very likely the reason RYR actually works to lower cholesterol. Now RYR products can only contain very slight traces of this statin and likely do not have the same effectiveness.[1]

2) LAVENDER OIL – It is suspected that Lavender oil works because it is a mood enhancer that relieves stress. But many natural essential oils do have a much more direct biochemical effect on the human body and it may well turn out that lavender oil does as well.[1]

3) CYPRESS OIL – Cypress oil has been linked to improved circulation and for that alone it comes highly recommended.[1]

4) ROSEMARY OIL – This essential oil has been linked to heart health and it is also known to be a strong and rather unique antioxidant as well and both of these roles are why it has been shown to lower cholesterol.[1]

5) BASIL – Many herbs both dried as well as fresh contain a host of powerful remedial compounds as well as essential nutrients including basil. I use it both dried and fresh when available in my oil and vinegar dressing.[1]

7) GINGER – Ginger is currently under investigation to verify claims that it can help lower cholesterol. It would come as no surprise because ginger is one of nature's most powerful remedial plants and it is also a very tasty spice. Ginger tea has been used in the far eastern countries for centuries to treat and cure just about every conceivable affliction and it may indeed have these amazing curative powers. By the way, don't count on Ginger ale to help you at all; they haven't used real ginger root to make that nuisance soda pop for over half a century.[1]

8) TURMERIC – This is another superfood spice with legendary antioxidant and anti-mutagenic powers (helps prevent damage to DNA in our cells) and is suspected of everything from being an effective treatment for some forms of cancer to being capable of lowering cholesterol. And the scientific community is taking it seriously because Turmeric is currently under investigation for many of its claimed powers.[1]

9) ALMONDS – These as well as PECANS and PISTACIOS are likely getting their power to lower cholesterol from their Omega-3 fatty acid ALA content. However, many nuts have various amounts of other essential nutrients in them including Vitamin E and minerals that are lacking in most folks daily diet that might also be playing a significant role in helping to lower cholesterol. Seeds and nuts are also high in quality fiber and they are all recommended. All seeds and nuts are definitely on the menu although sunflower seeds and walnuts should be at the top of your list for fighting cholesterol.[33]

10) LENTILS – These little legumes are high in fiber as well as copper. They are one of the few natural whole foods that have copper in high enough quantities in a pure natural form that is safe and can satisfy our daily requirements of it. Lentils are definitely on the menu for helping fight cholesterol.[34]

11) CHICK PEAS (GARBANZOS) – This is another legume that is loaded with fiber as well as copper and Vitamin B9 – FOLIC ACID. Mashed with a little olive oil creates HUMMUS which is one of the few natural food dips that is actually good for you.[35]

12) GRAPEFRUIT (and all other citrus fruits) – I hesitate to mention grapefruit because a lot of people are taking blood pressure medications as well as cholesterol medications and many of these are MAO Inhibitors and grapefruit is prohibited because it too is a powerful MAO Inhibitor which is EXACTLY WHY it is so good for you but not if you are already taking powerful MAOI's. Personally I would prefer to eat grapefruit which is NATURAL rather than take some highly concentrated drug that basically does the same thing, but grapefruit is natural and includes a substance that facilitates the burning of fat tissue (a dieter's best friend) AND they are loaded with water soluble fiber (the best kind especially for fighting cholesterol) AND they bring a lot of natural L-ascorbic acid a.k.a. pure true Vitamin C (as opposed to manufactured forms that are only 50% natural L-ascorbic acid and the other half is suspected of being TOXIC.) It is up to you, but if you are serious about changing your diet and your lifestyle then those harsh drugs may no longer be necessary and the grapefruit is an all-natural alternative that can and will do the job of many of those drugs. Although most of the other citrus fruits do not contain the strong MAOI concentrations and none have the fat burning enzyme, they are still loaded with water soluble fiber and Vitamin C and are definitely on the menu (people taking MAOI drugs must still check with their doctor before eating any citrus.)[36]

13) OLIVES and OLIVE OIL – I don't recommend going overboard with any vegetable oil especially store bought brands other than those they say they have only been filtered because they are all high in Omega-6 fatty acids. As your intake of these goes up, the effectiveness of the Omega-3's GOES DOWN: it is the ratio of the two that is critical. A diet high in Omega-6's – vegetable oils which are also found in NUTS – and low in Omega-3's can and will lead to high cholesterol. Because SEEDS and NUTS which are high in Omega-6's are already part of the plan, you will need to keep olives and olive oil to a minimum and monitor your intake of the Omega-6's to make sure that the Omega-3's outnumber them by at least 2 to 1 and higher is always better. Nevertheless olive oil has been shown to increase HDL, the "good" cholesterol levels in the blood and a dab in the salad dressing, or some hummus, is acceptable. Since Olives and Olive Oil have been shown to lower cholesterol, this is one of the few exceptions to the rule of avoiding vegetable oils.[1][37]

ROUNDING OUT THE ESSENTIAL NUTRIENTS

1) PHOSPHORUS – If you stick to the sunflower seed kernels you will get all of the phosphorus and selenium you need as well as a good dozes of Vitamins B1, B5 and E. Sunflower seed kernels are a TRUE SUPERFOOD and in my Top Recommended Superfoods list in "Vol. 5 – The Superfoods and Reading Nutrition Labels."[38]

2) MANGANESE AND COPPER – These trace essential nutrients are found in abundance in seeds and nuts so the sunflower seeds bring you most of what you need as do the Pumpkin seeds.[39][40]

3) ZINC – While the Pumpkin seeds are included primarily to give you a good boost of Zinc, alone they probably won't be enough. Just 1 oz. of canned wild oysters (most brands are wild "caught") will provide about 170% RDA of this valuable mineral linked to dozens of enzymes throughout the body. One ounce every other day will keep you right on top of your Zinc. I add them to my clam chowder so they "disappear" into there.[41]

4) CHLORINE – You will get all you need from the 1 teaspoon of IODIZED SALT daily. Chlorine is used in some electrolytic actions (like the sodium and potassium are as well) and is needed by the stomach to replenish its hydrochloric acid.[42]

5) CHOLINE – This one is a very BIG PROBLEM. It is almost exclusively found in fatty animal products like beef liver which is very high in cholesterol and not on the menu. Atlantic Mackerel, your #1 fish of choice because of its very high concentrations of Omega-3 fatty acids is definitely on the menu and a 4 to 5 ounce serving brings you about half of your daily requirement of choline. But the fish brings a lot of cholesterol and this is why you need the additional shot of Cod Liver Oil, 1 tablespoon per day, is highly recommended to help counteract these high cholesterol foods that are part of the diet (the oily fish.) Because you will be falling short of the mark with Choline you will need a good supplement. Most include 550mg which is the 100% RDA requirement so you might also want to try to find a supplement that provides about half of this (275mg) per pill or simply cut the pills in half because the Mackerel will bring you about half of what you need on a daily basis. Remember that Choline is a precursor to most of the B vitamins and has even been referred to sometimes as Vitamin B4 although this is not universally accepted. And you need a HUGE amount of it on a daily basis: 550mg. Compare that to Vitamin B3 Niacin which is needed in a much larger amount than most of the other B vitamins and we only need 20mg of it daily. For those with very high cholesterol or simply want to avoid the oily fish you will have to shop around online in order to find a natural extract Choline supplement.[43]

END OF CHAPTER QUIZ
1. Due to strict FDA regulations, which natural cholesterol treatment likely has far lower effectiveness than it used to?
    A. Lavender essential oil
    B. Turmeric
    C. Red Yeast Rice
    D. All of the above
    Answer: C. RYR used to contain significant amounts of a statin drug, likely naturally produced by the red yeast. The FDA watches these products and no longer allows them to contain any more than trace amounts of this substance which has likely lowered their effectiveness.
2. One of the most difficult B vitamins to get in sufficient quantities on a daily basis is:
    A. Vitamin B12
    B. Vitamin B3
    C. Vitamin B5
    D. Choline
    Answer: D. Choline is not a true B vitamin but the other B vitamins are made by starting with the choline molecule. We need a HUGE amount of choline on a daily basis and it is mostly found in high cholesterol foods like fish and eggs which should be avoided while correcting high cholesterol.
3. Many herbs, spices and their essential oils contain:
    A. High concentrations of unique phytonutrients
    B. High concentrations of antioxidants
    C. Powerful phytonutrients yet to be clinically tested
    D. All of the above
    Answer: D. Science has only just begun to investigate the compounds in your kitchen spice rack. Many common spices contain powerful antioxidants and unique phytonutrients currently being investigated for their potential health benefits.

At this point the strategy is complete so this chapter is a quick and complete recap of everything you need to do to take control, not only of your cholesterol, which is a SYMPTOM of deeper issues, but of your overall health as well.

The number one reason why the powerful and dangerous statin drugs control high cholesterol and yet the patient DIES, is very likely because the patient has made NO EFFORT to change their lifestyle away from what was causing the high cholesterol and basically killing them slowly in the first place. Taking the statin drugs (like Lipitor – since discontinued because too many patients died while taking it) to force lower cholesterol while continuing to pursue a deadly lifestyle of no exercise and continuing to eat terrible foods, is a recipe for disaster. Lack of exercise and poor diet are the number one killers of Americans and indeed all people worldwide regardless of their cholesterol levels, so in essence a person who will not do any exercise and who continues to eat a diet high in trash calories, saturated fats, cholesterol and artificial chemical cancer-causing additives while taking statins will certainly die early, but they will have good cholesterol levels, for whatever that will be worth at the funeral.

Sorry to be so blunt about it, but this book's title is "The TRUTH about...," not "Mollycoddle and politically correct pandering about..." Fix the CAUSES of the high cholesterol issues and they will simply go away. It is as simple as that. If your car won't start because the battery is dead, you can push it then jam it in gear and get it started. That will get you to the MECHANIC, or the parts store where you can either get your battery charged back up, or replace it. When my car reaches the point that the spark plugs and cables are so bad that the car won't even start, I have to spray the carburetor with starter fluid, and sometimes it won't stay running, but I am not going to rig up a can of starter fluid to feed the carburetor for the rest of my car's life. I am going to FIX the PROBLEM and replace the spark plugs and cables as quickly as possible because the starter fluid burns much hotter than regular gasoline and it will destroy the engine a lot faster. The same thing is happening to the people who take the statin drugs and refuse to FIX the CAUSE of the high cholesterol: the CAUSE remains and it will kill them.

Of course, if you are reading this book then I assume that you are serious about FIXING the problem rather than getting addicted to prescription drugs for the rest of your life. Over the past 20 years I have known a lot of people who suck down fistfuls of pills all day long and not one of these people has actually ever been CURED of their afflictions. Instead, they usually get a new pill or two ADDED to their suitcase sized pill organizers that they carry around all day so they can suck them down by the bucket load. No one gets CURED any more because cures don't create lifelong addicts and drug PUSHERS don't want their addicted customers to stop coming back for more either. This strategy will involve supplements, but I am assuming that you know that you have high cholesterol and you want to FIX the problem by throwing every weapon possible at it: you want a quick and decisive victory NOW; you want a CURE, not a lifetime of TREATMENTS also known as ADDICTION.

For those born with diabetes, I feel for them because the cure has been truly elusive, but for those who acquired Type II or "Late onset" diabetes, I have no pity for them, because they spent a lifetime sucking down GARBAGE FOOD until it made them sick and now they suck down a ton of GARBAGE medications and they STILL WON'T make any effort to correct their lifestyle. Some people I suppose are literally "stubborn until it kills them."

So let's go over the basic plan, then get into the details:

1) EXERCISE: Minimum 1 hour of aerobics. This does not mean engaging in movement like walking one block under an umbrella. If that is all you can do to start, then by all means do that, but aerobics means breathing hard and sweating and I know many people could never do that right off the bat, but you will have to work up to being able to do that for one hour a day. That can and will save your heart and therefore you, from an early grave.

2) NO MORE GARBAGE FOOD – The garbage food put you in the trouble you are now in, so there is no need to continue with it. Remember that the garbage food manufacturers are fully aware that they are sugar/saturated fat PUSHERS. Since they can't make donuts out of sugar and PIG LARD any more, they now fry them up in FAKE MANUFACTURED PIG LARD a.k.a. HYDROGENATED SOYBEAN OIL which is TOXIC to your liver: it is actually WORSE FOR YOU THAN THE PIG LARD! Soda pop and, by far the worst; all forms of alcohol MUST BE STOPPED. Beer has more sugar in it than soda pop. That's why they make it with hops, a plant whose leaves are about as bitter as aspirin, to try to cover all of that sugar. Even distilled spirits are loaded with sugar and they all mess with your liver and will make it diseased and that disease can kill you and one of the early warning signs that it is getting sick and going to kill you is high cholesterol.

3) PROPER NUTRITIOUS DIET – Start eating foods that are good for you exclusively. Good food is good medicine. And bad food is as deadly as rattlesnake venom; the only difference is how long it takes to kill you, but they both will kill you. And the failure of people in modern times to fully appreciate this is astounding. You certainly wouldn't ever decide that you are sick and tired of breathing plain old nitrogen and oxygen air and decide that from now on, all you are ever going to breathe is pure sulfur hexafluoride. As horrifying as the name sounds, it is actually a very stable, clear, inert gas, but it has no value to you either, so you will suffocate to death a few minutes after you make this change. Everybody gets that, but they don't get the idea that eating GARBAGE all day every day is just as deadly, it just takes twenty to thirty years to kill you, but it does: over 700,000 people DIE each year in the United States from heart attacks and cancer, and almost all of those deaths are being caused by the GARBAGE the food manufacturers are peddling to their addicts.

Now for the details…

DAILY DIET

1) BREAKFAST – OLD-FASHIONED OATMEAL. Add 1 oz. WALNUTS, 2oz RAISINS, 2 oz. WHEAT GERM, 1 tablespoon CINNAMON, ½ teaspoon of IODIZED SALT or SEA SALT, and sweeten with raw BEE HONEY. This breakfast is loaded with Fiber, Manganese, Molybdenum, Omega-3 alpha-Linoleic acid, Vitamin B9 – Folate, Sodium, Iodine, Iron and Chromium (in the raisins,) and cinnamon has dozens of phytonutrients in it and has been shown in clinical trials to be effective in helping regulate proper blood sugar levels. It also has an ORAC (Oxygen Radical Absorption Capacity) Score of over 130,000 making it 185 TIMES stronger in antioxidant potential than raw carrots. Drink 12 oz. LOW SODIUM V-8 (or equivalent vegetable juice of any other brand.) This will provide about 36% percent of your daily requirement of Potassium. Finish up with 1 BANANA (another 14% Potassium)[44] and one whole GRAPEFRUIT with no sugar added (I let them slightly over-ripen and peel and eat like an orange.) It is low calorie and provides over 100% RDA of Vitamin C plus it has been shown in studies to help people lose weight.

2) LUNCH – Tossed green salad: LETTUCE, SPINACH, PEELED CUCUMBER, ONIONS, RADISHES, GREEN BELL PEPPER, ARUGULA, KALE, HOMEMADE OIL AND VINEGAR DRESSING. Be sure to include some spinach or kale or both at the very least. ½ cup of either will provide you with well over 100% RDA of Vitamin K. The Homemade Oil and Vinegar is: 1 cup Extra Virgin Olive Oil (although I sometimes use the cheaper lighter one) to which you should add: FRESH or DRIED BASIL, OREGANO, BLACK PEPPER, PAPRIKA, CILANTRO, SAGE, ROSEMARY, and fresh minced GARLIC. Then add RED WINE VINEGAR to taste. Let stand for one day and use about 1 to 2 tablespoons in your salad. You can also add 2 oz. PARMESAN/ROMANO CHEESE into the salad. While this does bring calories it also brings about 60% of your daily requirement of Calcium (one of the densest sources of Calcium of any food.) The Olive Oil has been shown to help reduce cholesterol, the Vinegar has been shown to lower blood pressure, all of those spices have been shown to support cardiovascular health and they all have astronomical ORAC Scores as well (super-powerful antioxidants, so the more the merrier!) Even with the Olive oil and the Parmesan cheese, this is a rather low calorie lunch.

3) DINNER – This one is up to you, but ideally it should include 4 oz. of any fish (Atlantic Mackerel, Wild-caught Salmon, Tuna, Cod, Sardines are the top choices in that order.) Preferably baked if purchased raw. Sides: Green peas, Lentils, Chickpeas, Blackeye peas, Turnips, Beets, Squash (any variety from Acorn to Butternut, to Yellow to Winter) Green beans (lightly steamed and still crispy) Cabbage, Broccoli, Cauliflower, Carrots, Spinach; Turnip, Collard or Mustard Greens, Zucchini, Okra, Bok Choy, Shallots, Napa cabbage (all preferably steamed.) Add any of these to boiled vegetables: Black Pepper, Garlic, Onions, Chives, Oregano, Basil, Paprika, Parsley, Cilantro, Sage, Rosemary, Cloves, Turmeric. Garnish with melted real Swiss cheese, butter, Parmesan/Romano cheese, Homemade oil and vinegar dressing, sour cream (it is dairy and FAR HEALTHIER than mayonnaise and its kin – see Foods to Avoid below.)

4) DESERTS – FRUITS with a preference for: apples (fresh white pulp only, brown has lost a lot of its antioxidant potential) bananas, apricots, blueberries, blackberries, mulberries (these three berries are loaded with anthocyanidins – powerful antioxidants) pineapple, guava, citrus. YOGURT, preferably organic.

5) SNACKS – 100% Pure "Unsweetened Baker's Chocolate" bars dipped in raw bee Honey, Celery, Carrots, Raisins, Sunflower Seed Kernels, Pumpkin seeds.

7) SOUP – Add this side dish to lunch salad or dinner: Ready-To-Eat New England Clam Chowder, but add a ½ can of chopped clams and 1 oz (1/8 can) of boiled oysters. Real Chicken Soup: boil skinned chicken and add turmeric and any other spices and veggies from the approved list above that you choose.

8) DRINKS – 24 oz per day of 100% Pure Concord Grape Juice, 32 oz per day of Low Sodium V-8 (or any other brand as long as they have used potassium salt to make it salty flavored.) Cranberry Juice, Pomegranate Juice (these last two are loaded with antioxidants, Pomegranates have the second highest ORAC Score of fresh fruits (over 55,000) and you should juice your own, you can juice them just like oranges on the same apparatus.)

9) SPICE RACK –

Starting with the **CINNAMON**, all of these have very high ORAC Scores meaning they have antioxidant potentials dozens to hundreds of times higher than raw carrots. which are loaded with beta-carotene; a very powerful antioxidant. Cinnamon is also linked to proper insulin utilization by the body and is a critical part of keeping the blood sugar system under control and to avoid diabetes.[22]

TURMERIC – contains curcumin and there is mounting evidence that this may be an effective treatment for CANCER as well as a very effective preventative of this dreaded malady.[45]

GARLIC – Contains over 40 identified glucosinolates (sulfur containing compounds) including Allicin which gives garlic its unique aroma and flavor and is believed to be the "active ingredient" that causes it to lower the cholesterol levels in the blood and to also lower blood pressure.[4]

OREGANO – has a huge ORAC Score and contains carvacrol known for its antibacterial power but also under investigation for its many other potential health benefits including prevention and treatment of cancer.[46]

SAGE – very high ORAC Score and contains Carnosol and Perillyl alcohol both under investigation for their potential cancer fighting power as possible future treatments of some forms of this terrible disease.[47]

ROSEMARY – contains Carnasol and Betulinic acid which has known anti-inflammatory properties as well as anti-cancer power.[49]

CLOVES – Contains a host of phytonutrients including Eugenol and has one of the highest ORAC Scores for any readily available spice (over 290,000) and for that alone it is well worth it to add to your cooking, but the health advantages of cloves are astounding, it is antibacterial (able to kill many oral and gastrointestinal infections,) is a strong liver tonic (helps the liver resist oxidative stress and function better) an anti-mutagen (protects cell's DNA from being damaged by toxins) assists insulin pathways (helps blood sugar regulation and may prevent diabetes) and the list goes on.[50]

BLACK PEPPER – Contains Piperine and traces of Capsaicin (the heat in hot peppers) and early research is suggesting that this common spice (best from a peppercorn grinder) is not only a powerful antioxidant but also an antibacterial, helps regulate blood sugar, kills colon cancer cells, assists the digestive process by stimulating the production of stomach acid AND the absorption of various nutrients by the intestines including such other powerful phytonutrients as curcumin found in Turmeric. So add a heavy dash of black pepper into every dish that is getting a blast of the other spices to help your body absorb all of their nutrients even better.[51]

PAPRIKA – This dried finely ground red pepper powder has an impressive array of phytonutrients including beta-carotene beta-cryptoxanthin, zeaxanthin, lutein, and capsaicin to name just a few. Paprika has an impressive ORAC Score of nearly 22000 and aside from the usual effects of helping blood sugar levels and serving as an anti-carcinogen, it is being investigated for its very powerful anti-inflammatory effects and it is believed that it may help treat autoimmune disorders including arthritis.[52]

9) OTHER: Add toasted whole wheat bread (no more than two slices per day) to breakfast, lunch or dinner. For lunch or dinner I turn it into garlic toast by heating butter and a teaspoon of minced garlic and drizzling it onto the toast. For breakfast I just add a little butter and cinnamon (most jams and jellies are loaded with every conceivable chemical as well as that ubiquitous BANE "High fructose corn syrup" or worse; some miserable SOY by-product and both are to be avoided…

FOODS TO AVOID

While correcting your cholesterol levels you must avoid the following:

1) PACKAGED AND/OR PROCESSED FOODS including100% Whole Grain bread. Get this from the local bakery with NO ADDED CHEMICALS, NO HIGH FRUCTOSE CORN SYRUP, and ABSOLUTELY NEVER any HYDROGENATED (or "hydrolyzed") VEGETABLE OIL of any kind. All three of these along with processed white cane sugar are PROVEN irritants of the liver that can and do cause diabetes and CANCER.

2) NO SOY or its BY-PRODUCTS: these are CHEAP GARBAGE FILLERS in virtually all processed and packaged foods that they won't even feed to cows, goats or pigs. If it's not even good enough for them, what are they doing giving it to us? Many studies are starting to show that chronic overindulgence in soy beans and their by-products can be TOXIC to humans and this CRUD is DEFINITELY TOXIC to grazing animals: enough said. If you are drinking soy milk I urge you to consider Almond milk or some other alternative.

3) NO "FORTIFIED" or "ENRICHED" foods. The added vitamins and minerals are always synthetic and inferior quality; some are actually BAD for you.

4) NO STARCHY FOODS: This means no potatoes or their kin: sweet potatoes (even though they are very high in nutritional value) yucca, malanga, boniato, etc. No GRAINS other than what I have already allowed so no: CORN, RICE, etc.

5) NO BEANS other than the legumes I have already listed as "OK" so no: Pinto beans, Lima beans, Kidney beans, Black beans, Navy beans, etc. All of these are high in a bad form of fiber which is what makes them ahem… "Difficult to digest." Some do have a lot of nutrients in them but they are just not worth it.

6) EGGS and all of their products. Until you have fixed your cholesterol it is best to avoid all foods made from eggs including most baked goods and all forms of pasta. (I sorely miss my pasta, and I cheat and have it ONCE a month.)

6) MAYONNAISE and its KIN: this includes creamy store bought salad dressings and creamy dips which are all made with raw egg which is BAD FOR YOU. Raw egg binds with Vitamin B7 – Biotin in particular but it also blocks the absorption of all B vitamins to some extent: you don't need this slime in your digestive tract BLOCKING the absorption of all of the B Vitamins that you NEED and are PAYING FOR and PAYING ATTENTION TO specifically in order to get them. Drop these foods forever.

50

7) PORK and PROCESSED meats: No: hotdogs, sausages, bacon, "luncheon meat" (i.e. "Spam") "potted meat" (i.e. "Deviled Ham") etc. I have no quarrel with jerky and kippered meat except that most modern packaged products add NITRITES as preservatives and these are DREADFUL POISONS to the liver. Pork is the bottom of the barrel as far as meat quality goes. I have it once a month now, but I am sticking strictly to this natural whole food regimen as well.

WHAT DOES THIS MENU BRING?

Its all fine and dandy but in the end you should keep in mind that this menu is MEDICINAL; it is set up to LOWER CHOLESTEROL and triglyceride levels and to return the BALANCE to the proper proportions of all three (LDL's, HDL's and triglycerides) in the blood. It is also designed around low calorie foods and the only foods that bring cholesterol are the oily fish but they also bring the much needed Omega-3's so they are worth it. Nevertheless, you should also keep in mind which foods are bringing which needed nutrients.[1]

VITAMIN A – 1 carrot, Raw = 200% RDA, cooked: 100% RDA[53]

VITAMIN B1 (Thiamine) – ½ cup Sunflower Seed Kernels: 100% RDA.[54]

VITAMIN B2 (Riboflavin) – Covered in the next chapter.[55]

VITAMIN B3 (Niacin) – Covered in the next chapter.[14]

CHOLINE – Covered in the next chapter.[43]

VITAMIN B5 (Pantothenic acid) – ½ cup sunflower seeds.[57]

VITAMIN B6 (Pyridoxine) – Covered in the next chapter.[58]

VITAMIN B7 (Biotin) – 2 Slices of Whole Grain Bread which also brings BETAINE, an amino acid that helps lower homocysteine levels in the blood which is directly linked to lowering plaque build up on arterial walls (atherosclerosis) which leads to heart attack and stroke.[59]

VITAMIN B9 (Folate) – The Whole Grain Bread, Wheat germ and chickpeas cover this vitamin easily.[60]

VITAMIN B12 (Methylcobalamin) – 100% RDA in 3 oz sardines or Atlantic mackerel. Covered in the next chapter.[61]

VITAMIN C – The grapefruit brings about 150% RDA.[62]

VITAMIN D3 (cholecalciferol) – Covered in the next chapter.[24]

VITAMIN E – ½ cup sunflower seeds and the wheat germ take care of this in excess of 100% RDA.[26]

VITAMIN K – The spinach or kale in the lunch salad has this thoroughly covered.[21]

CALCIUM – 1 x 8 oz cup of milk brings about 30% RDA. 1 oz. of Parmesan/Romano cheese also brings about 30% RDA, 1 oz, Swiss cheese brings about 20% RDA. Just make sure it all adds up to 100% RDA at the end of the day.[23]

CHLORINE – 1 teaspoon of SEA SALT or IODIZED SALT per day while making sure that you are NOT getting Sodium from any other food source (they do sneak it into cheeses.)[42]

51

CHROMIUM – 24 oz. 100% Concord Grape Juice will bring 100% of this critical mineral. Slightly more than 1 cup of broccoli also brings 100% RDA of Chromium and 1 teaspoon of garlic brings 12% RDA. Be sure to get those 100% RDA of this mineral which helps the body use insulin and therefore helps straighten out blood sugar issues and also helps prevent diabetes. The grape juice also brings Resveratrol: known for its powers to suppress at least three compounds in the body that promote aging and thus it is an anti-aging nutrient, Myricetin: research has just begun on this miraculous compound that is BOTH a powerful antioxidant AND a powerful OXIDANT AT THE SAME time! It relieves oxidative stress throughout the body AND helps destroy invading viruses. Anthocyanidins: potent antioxidants.[19]

COPPER – Easily covered by the ½ cup sunflower seeds and the oatmeal and wheat germ.[40]

IODINE – 1 teaspoon of SEA SALT or IODIZED SALT per day while making sure that you are NOT getting Sodium from any other food source (they do sneak it into cheeses.)[16]

IRON – 2.5 oz Canned Wild Clams bring 100% RDA of this critical mineral that is HARD to get in this amount by most other foods. The 4 oz. Dark Chocolate ALSO BRING 100% RDA. So eat ONE or the OTHER on a daily basis. I alternate my soup with my salad, one day it is clam chowder, the next it is homemade chicken and vegetable soup. So desert after the chicken soup lunch is the 4 oz bar of dark chocolate.[32]

MAGNESIUM – 4 oz. 100% Pure Dark Chocolate brings 100% RDA.[20]

MANGANESE – Easily covered by the ½ cup sunflower seeds and the oatmeal and wheat germ.[39]

MOLYBDENUM – Easily covered by the Oatmeal, but green peas and chickpeas are loaded with it too.[63]

PHOSPHORUS – ½ cup sunflower seed kernels takes care of this easily.[38]

POTASSIUM – 32 oz. Low Sodium V-8 solves this problem and it is a BIG POBLEM. You can drink all of that V-8 or add bananas which cover about 14% RDA each.[27]

SELENIUM – ½ cup sunflower seed kernels (now you begin to see why they are worth it (about 4 oz.) because they solve FIVE essential nutrients easily.)[18]

SODIUM – 1 teaspoon of SEA SALT or IODIZED SALT per day while making sure that you are NOT getting Sodium from any other food source (they do sneak it into cheeses.)[27]

SULFUR – There is no RDA for this essential mineral, but they assume that most people with diversified natural whole food diet are getting plenty. Cabbage, Broccoli, Cauliflower, Garlic and onions are loaded with sulfur and on the menu.[64]

ZINC – Just 1 oz of canned wild oysters brings about 170% of this critical mineral. It takes about 5 oz. of pumpkin seeds (which are very light and occupy over 2 liquid cups in volume) to bring 100% RDA. 1 oz. of oysters every other day plus just 1 oz. of pumpkin seeds daily will keep you on course with this essential nutrient that promotes immune system health.[41]

OMEGA-3 Fatty Acids – 1 oz Walnuts yields about 2600mg ALA, 4 oz. of Atlantic Mackerel yields 4000mg EPA and DHA.[15]

"NET NEGATIVE CALORIE" FOODS – Other than the meats, grains, seeds and nuts, almost all of the vegetables and fruits are relatively low calorie foods that are excellent for your health.[65]

SPICE RACK – An impressive array of phytonutrients including some of the most powerful antioxidants by weight. 5 to 6 grams of clove powder (a heaping teaspoon) has the antioxidant power of 5 POUNDS of raw carrots. Most have distinctive phytonutrients with well documented positive health benefits and are currently under investigation for their powers ranging from antibacterial, to anti-inflammatory to powerful cancer fighting agents that might end up being used as very effective cancer treatments in the future.[66]

END OF CHAPTER QUIZ

1. Which food provides the 100% RDA requirements for no less than FIVE different essential nutrients?
A. Sea Salt
B. Atlantic Mackerel
C. Dark Chocolate
D. Sunflower Seed Kernels
Answer: D. About 4 oz. provide 100% RDA of Vitamins B1, B5 and E as well as Phosphorus and Selenium.

2. Which of the following will provide 100% RDA of three essential minerals and only takes 1 teaspoon to do it?
A. Sea Salt
B. Atlantic Mackerel
C. Dark Chocolate
D. Sunflower Seed Kernels
Answer: A. 1 teaspoon of Sea Sat provides you with at least 100% RDA of Sodium (it is NEEDED) Chlorine and Iodine which is very difficult to find in most natural whole foods.

3. Which of the following foods has the highest concentration of DHA and EPA Omega-3 fatty acids?
A. Sea Salt
B. Atlantic Mackerel
C. Dark Chocolate
D. Sunflower Seed Kernels
Answer: B. Atlantic Mackerel has the highest content of DHA and EPA of any commonly available natural whole food.

In addition to a healthy natural whole foods diet, you will need to augment that with a carefully selected group of supplements that will shore up some of the essential nutrients that are either coming up short in your natural whole foods choices or that bring way too many calories, saturated fats and cholesterol to be of use while trying to control your cholesterol levels. First amongst these is CHOLINE, which is normally found in fatty high cholesterol foods.

THE SUPPLEMENTS YOU WILL NEED

1) CHOLINE – Because this is a very important nutrient related to all of the other B vitamins and the liver can make some of the B Vitamins out of Choline, it is important to get 100% RDA of it and it is usually only found in foods high in saturated fat and cholesterol like Beef Liver and Eggs. Since you want to cut down on the consumption of both saturated fats and cholesterol, then you will have to find a quality Choline supplement and one made from natural food extract should be your top priority. Most bring 550mg per pill which is the 100% RDA amount that you need.[43]

2) VITAMIN A (RETINOL) – 1 Tablespoon of Cod Liver Oil will provide about 100% of this important vitamin.[53]

3) VITAMIN B2 (RIBOFLAVIN) – While this essential Vitamin can be found in many common foods, it is usually not enough to meet the 100% RDA requirement of it. A natural food extract is a priority over manufactured synthetic forms which are the only ones found on the shelves of most stores other than specialty stores.[55]

4) VITAMIN B3 (NIACIN) – This one is CRITICAL to the plan to lower cholesterol because this vitamin converts the bad LDL cholesterol into the good HDL cholesterol and most doctors recommend taking the supplement for this reason. Find a quality natural food extract product offering 20mg pills (100% RDA amount per pill) and take a minimum of three per day, one with each meal although I have found sources recommending up to 1000% RDA daily, this is likely excessive and your body will very likely get Niacin flushes in the skin (prickly sensation) which means it is not being used and will just get removed by the kidneys anyway. Nevertheless you should try to take four or five of those pills per day and stop when you get the niacin flush which means it is being wasted at that point. Try to space them out evenly during the day and accompany them with meals or substantial snacks.[14]

5) VITAMIN B6 (PYRIDOXINE) – Another Vitamin that is not easy to get in 100% RDA amounts daily from natural whole foods. Rather than fret over it, just find a quality natural food extract and take as directed to get 100% RDA of this essential Vitamin.[58]

6) VITAMIN B12 (METHYLCOBALAMIN) – This is the animal B vitamin and it is deeply involved in proper brain function like all of the other B vitamins, but this one is almost only found in animal foods and not plants. I strongly recommend that you do NOT take a Vitamin B Complex because these are invariably made from manufactured synthetic versions of all of those B vitamins and SYNTHETIC B12 is NOT the same molecule (Cyanocobalamin) as the naturally occurring one in animal foods and our own brains (Methylcobalamin.) There are many natural food extract Vitamin B12 products on the market, but I have not found one in any big store.[61]

7) VITAMIN D3 (CHOLECALCIFEROL) – 1 Tablespoon of Cod Liver Oil will provide 150% RDA of this natural form vitamin.[24]

8) MAGNESIUM – On the days when you eat 4 oz. of Pure 100% Cacao dark chocolate (Unsweetened Baker's Chocolate) you will also get about 100% RDA of this critical mineral. On the other days you should take "Chelated Magnesium."[20]

9) OMEGA-3 DHA/EPA – 1 Tablespoon of Cod Liver Oil will provide about 2600mg of these vital nutrients that are at the center of the plan to lower cholesterol. This should be taken in addition to eating fish. If you do not like or want to eat fish daily, then the Cod Liver Oil is essential.[15]

10) FISH OIL – In addition to the Cod Liver Oil you should also take at least 1000mg of Fish Oil supplement with it. If you do not plan to eat fish then you will need to take 1000mg with each meal as well. So you are getting 2600mg of DHA and EPA from the Cod Liver Oil and an additional 3000mg from the pills. The goal is to make sure you get much more Omega-3 in your daily diet than Omega-6's (found in vegetable oils, seeds and nuts.) With this regimen you should skip the walnuts altogether because they are very high in Omega-6's.[1]

11) GARLIC – Avoid products that are "odorless" because the Allicin is gone and it may be one of the active ingredients that helps the garlic to lower the bad LDL's and raise the good HDL's. Think of odorless garlic as a de-clawed cat (not going to get much hunting done!) Take about 500mg per day. There is some skepticism in the scientific community about the efficacy of garlic but even the skeptics say it does reduce cholesterol by 10%.[4]

12) CoQ10 – This is very heart friendly. Take as directed until your cholesterol levels show significant improvement then taper off.[1]

13) MILK THISTLE – This is very important for the plan to work (everything is really!) There are a bunch of phytonutrients in Milk Thistle including Silymarin and dozens of closely related compounds called "Stilbenoids" and these work like liver tonic helping the liver to detoxify and repair itself. The reason you have high cholesterol and why it persists long after you give up a diet of toxic foods and alcohol and so on, is because the liver is beat up by all of that abuse and it is constantly working 24/7 on the vast array of molecules in every meal you eat. The silymarin can help it get back to OPTIMUM THRIVE-LEVEL health. Take only as directed because this one is powerful medicine and you should never overdo it with curative plants like this one that have a very well known and documented powerful effect on the body. (More is NEVER BETTER when it comes to powerful medications which can quickly turn TOXIC in excess.)[8]

MORE CONCERNING THE OMEGA-3's

The Omega-3's are FATTY ACIDS that are dissolved in fish fats and oils in the Cod Liver OIL and the Fish OIL pills. Fats and Oils are difficult to absorb in the intestines and difficult to handle in the liver. This is why it is critical to give the liver all of the help we can find for it. And that breakfast of Oatmeal and wheat germ is high in fiber which tends to cling to fats, oils and cholesterol and PREVENT their absorption. It is a dilemma since we WANT these particular oils to get absorbed and not scrubbed away by the fiber.

Also, there is ONE thing in the kitchen that helps the breakdown and absorption of fats and oils and will facilitate the absorption of the Cod Liver Oil and the Fish Oil pills: BLACK PEPPER. This is the main benefit of the spice due to its high concentrations of Piperine. Therefore the Cod Liver Oil and the Fish Oil pills need to be taken long after breakfast with a snack low in fiber and high in black pepper. You can decide for yourself how to proceed but my handy snack that helps with this is: squares of block cheese of any kind you like topped with small red tomato slices blackened with black pepper from a peppercorn grinder; quite tasty (and sneezy!) and loads up the intestines with the important black pepper which helps them absorb ALL of the nutrients in the Cod Liver Oil, the Fish Oil pills and the cheese (bringing a lot of Calcium to the party as well.)

MORE CONCERNING LIVER DETOX

The number one liver detoxifier is CHLOROPHYLL.[67] And you get this in superb quantity and quality from raw edible dark leafy greens and the most readily available to most folks is spinach in the produce section of your local grocery store. This is a MUST addition to your lunch salad because it brings a LOT of chlorophyll in natural LIVING healthy form and plenty of Vitamin K also in natural form. Canned spinach "No salt" is also good, but treat it like soup and empty the spice rack into it. Bring a small amount of water to boil and turn down the heat to just below boiling and add the spices. Simmer for five minutes then add the entire contents of the can and raise the heat until it just starts to boil vigorously and serve. Good choices are black pepper, turmeric, sage and rosemary.

Take the Milk Thistle pill any time during the day. The contents are basically dried leaf powder and the stilbenoids are readily absorbed by the intestines when the pill accompanies any substantial meal or snack.

AVOID B COMPLEX SUPPLEMENTS

You will be paying for B1, B5, B7 and B9 which is not necessary if you are following the basic dietary plan involving the Sunflower seed kernels (B1 and B5), the Whole Wheat Bread (B7) and Wheat Germ (B9). Furthermore, ALL B complex supplements that I have found so far include B12 as CYANOCOBALAMIN which is SYNTHETIC and NOT the same molecule as found in nature and our brains called METHYLCOBALAMIN. Since man is batting nearly a THOUSAND with making artificial additives to food that cause CANCER, I personally do want to roll the dice with my BRAIN to see if this stuff causes CANCER like everything else we cook up in our Frankenstein lab test tubes. Take time to search for and locate reputable vendors online selling natural extract individual supplements and buy each one that you actually need independently and take them together before a substantial meal. It will cost more, but the high quality of the Vitamins is WORTH it. Why PAY for vitamins only to get CANCER-causing, CHEAP SUBSTITUTES for the ones found in nature? Would you go to the doctor and pay him to GIVE you a disease? I think not.

I am not saying that these synthetics cause cancer, I am saying that the risk is there and there is ZERO RISK in taking natural extracted vitamins. I keep thinking about that number almost ¾ of a MILLION people die each year from heart attacks and CANCER and those numbers are not getting better; they are getting WORSE every year. There is little doubt that the global contamination of nuclear fallout started by the nuclear weapon tests in White Sands New Mexico during the Second World War, and the disasters at Chernobyl and Fukushima are largely to blame, but global contamination by DDT insecticide and the destruction of the ozone layer by hairspray contribute to this as well and the final component of this modern death epidemic is the CANCER COCKTAIL of artificial chemicals being ADDED to our foods.

Why ADD more ARTIFICIAL chemicals to your body in the form of FAKE vitamins? So a B complex at the nearest store costs $5 and EACH natural extract costs $10. They are all WELL WORTH it because you are buying vitamins that will HELP you with NO DOUBT, but those FAKE vitamins carry a risk with them and COULD kill you.

STAY THE COURSE

The liver regenerates on average in about 6 weeks. Statistically speaking, after about 12 weeks you have a whole new liver, all of the cells have been replaced by new ones. Of course this is an ongoing process so some will still be there from before the 3 month period began but most will be new ones born after the 3 month period began. To that end, you have a target time frame: 3 months. During that time frame you want to ease the stress on the liver, give it powerful natural medicine, and as much detoxifying agents as possible so that the NEW liver you will have 3 months from now will be far healthier, indeed at OPTIMUM THRIVE-LEVEL health.[68] And that NEW liver should be functioning properly making the correct amounts of the LDL's, HDL's and triglycerides IF you stick strictly to the plan.

DISCLAIMER AND WARNING

MOST IMPORTANTLY of all: you do NOT have to take my word for anything I have said in this book either. Take my recommendations to your DOCTOR or a certified nutrition specialist and verify everything. Many people have allergies and other digestive anomalies such as the inability to tolerate lactose in dairy products, gluten in wheat products, or to even properly digest fats and oils. Some people have early warning signs of kidney trouble which the doctor can easily identify from a blood sample and the diet I have laid out here could SEVERELY affect kidneys that are already on the brink. Incidentally, celery is one of the few potentially powerful kidney tonics (helps the kidneys detox and regenerate) known and I encourage everyone to eat as much as they can (a good "Net negative calorie" food that will fill your stomach and reduce the load of BAD foods you eat during the day) and to drink some water between all of the V-8 and Grape Juice, both of which are HARSH for the kidneys.

DO NOT MAKE ANY CHANGES TO YOUR DIET IF YOU ARE TAKING ANY MEDICATIONS INCLUDING BLOOD THINNERS OR MEDICATIONS FOR DIABETES, HIGH BLOOD PRESSURE, OR HIGH CHOLESTEROL. CONSULT YOUR DOCTOR FIRST.

END OF CHAPTER QUIZ

1. Most B complex supplements are bad primarily because:
 A. They include a purely synthetic version of Vitamin B12 which is not the same molecule as the one found in nature
 B. All of the B Vitamins in the complex are artificial, not natural
 C. Both A and B
 D. Neither A or B
 Answer: C. All of the B vitamins in most B Complex products that I have found contain only artificial versions of the vitamins and no natural extract source versions which are the only ones you should take.

2. 1 Tablespoon of Cod Liver Oil provides:
 A. 100% RDA of Vitamin A
 B. 2600mg of Omega-3 DHA and EPA
 C. 150% RDA Vitamin D3
 D. All of the above.
 Answer: D. That is exactly why it is so good for you even if it does taste dreadful.

3. One of the most important nutrients you need in relatively large quantities that is exclusively found in high amounts in high fat and high cholesterol foods is:
 A. Riboflavin
 B. Niacin
 C. Potassium

D. Choline

Answer: D. Choline is usually highest in fatty and high cholesterol foods like beef liver and eggs which are NOT on the menu while you are fixing your cholesterol issues.

4. The average healthy adult liver takes how long to fully regenerate (replace all cells with new ones)?

A. 27 weeks

B. 27 months

C. 27 days

D. The liver does not regenerate

Answer: B. The average healthy human liver regenerates in about 27 months. This is your target window of time. Spend the next 27 months doing everything RIGHT for your liver and overall health and avoiding ALL bad foods and alcohol to help the NEW liver you will have in 27 months be FAR healthier and this plan will work.

5. Because the spice rack is so loaded with very concentrated and powerful antioxidants and other phytonutrients which type of home cooked food is the best way to get ALL of what you add to the pot?

A. Boiled vegetables

B. Soups

C. Casseroles

D. Both B and C

Answer: D. Both B and C. Casseroles are solid and hold every grain of every spice you added to the dish anc soups are great because you consume the broth as well as the solids.

6. Which of the spices is so effective because it helps the digestive tract break down and absorb fats and all other nutrients in the foods in the meal?

A. Black pepper

B. Turmeric

C. Cinnamon

D. Sea Salt

Answer: A. Black pepper which is also a powerful antioxidant and is currently being investigated for many other health benefits.

7. Which mineral is needed in large amounts daily and should be supplemented in a chelated form?

A. Phosphorus.

B. Calcium

C. Sodium

D. Magnesium

Answer: D. We need about 400mg daily and the Chelate is by far the best form to take in a supplement.

THANK YOU AND GOD BLESS AND GOOD LUCK AND ABOVE ALL ELSE: TAKE CARE OF YOURSELF (BECAUSE NO ONE ELSE IS GOING TO DO IT)!

REFERENCES

Most information in this book was found at: wikipedia.org, nutritiondata.self.com, myfooddata.com, WebMD, draxe.com, whfoods.com, and the fda.gov and nih.gov. These websites are excellent resources and you should check them out.

[1] "How to Lower Cholesterol Naturally": https://draxe.com/lower-cholesterol-naturally-fast/ Retrieved on 9/18/18 * "Alternative Treatments for High Cholesterol" https://www.webmd.com/cholesterol-management/lower-cholesterol-9/supplement-herbs Reviewed by James Beckerman MD, Retrieved on 9/18/18

[2] Fiber: https://draxe.com/high-fiber-foods/ Retrieved on 8/20/18

[3] Oats: https://nutritiondata.self.com/facts/breakfast-cereals/1597/2 Retrieved on 9/12/18

[4] Garlic: https://www.webmd.com/vitamins/ai/ingredientmono-300/garlic Retrieved on 9/18/18

[5] Walnuts: https://nutritiondata.self.com/facts/nut-and-seed-products/3138/2 Retrieved on 9/12/18

[6] Atlantic Mackerel: https://nutritiondata.self.com/facts/finfish-and-shellfish-products/4072/2 Retrieved on 9/12/18

[7] The Nine Essential Amino Acids (Complete Protein): Rohini Nag, https://www.healthkart.com/connect/the-all-essential-amino-acids-foods-list-you-must-know-about/ Retrieved on 8/20/18

[8] Milk Thistle: Reviewed by Suzanne R. Steinbaum MD, https://www.webmd.com/digestive-disorders/milk-thistle-benefits-and-side-effects Retrieved on 9/25/18

[9] Sunflower seed kernels: https://nutritiondata.self.com/facts/nut-and-seed-products/3077/2 Retrieved on 9/12/18

[10] Carrots: https://nutritiondata.self.com/facts/vegetables-and-vegetable-products/2383/2 Retrieved on 9/12/18

[11] Celery: https://nutritiondata.self.com/facts/vegetables-and-vegetable-products/2396/2 Retrieved on 9/12/18

[12] Pumpkin seeds: https://nutritiondata.self.com/facts/nut-and-seed-products/3141/2 Retrieved on 9/12/18

[13] Dark chocolate: https://nutritiondata.self.com/facts/sweets/5390/2 Retrieved on 9/12/18

[14] Vitamin B3 – Niacin: https://draxe.com/niacin-side-effects/ Retrieved on 7/24/18 * https://www.myfooddata.com/articles/foods-high-in-niacin-vitamin-B3.php Retrieved on 7/24/18 * http://www.whfoods.com/genpage.php?tname=nutrient&dbid=83 Retrieved on 7/24/18

[15] Omega-3 fatty acids: https://draxe.com/omega-3-benefits-plus-top-10-omega-3-foods-list/ Retrieved on 8/23/18

[16] Iodine: https://draxe.com/iodine-rich-foods/ Retrieved on 7/26-18 * https://www.myfooddata.com/articles/natural-foods-high-in-iodine.php Retrieved on 7/26-18

[18] Selenium: https://draxe.com/selenium-foods/ Retrieved on 8/23/18 * https://www.myfooddata.com/articles/foods-high-in-selenium.php Retrieved on /8/23/18 * http://www.whfoods.com/genpage.php?tname=nutrient&dbid=95 Retrieved on 8/23/18

[19] Chromium: https://draxe.com/what-is-chromium/ Retrieved on 8/23/18 * http://www.whfoods.com/genpage.php?tname=nutrient&dbid=51 Retrieved on 8/23/18

[20] Magnesium: https://draxe.com/magnesium-deficient-top-10-magnesium-rich-foods-must-eating/ Retrieved on 7/30/18 * https://www.myfooddata.com/articles/foods-high-in-magnesium.php Retrieved on 7/30/18 * http://www.whfoods.com/genpage.php?tname=nutrient&dbid=75 Retrieved on 7/30/18

[21] Vitamin K: https://draxe.com/vitamin-k-deficiency/ Retrieved on 7/28/18 * https://www.myfooddata.com/articles/food-sources-of-vitamin-k.php Retrieved on 7/28/18 * http://www.whfoods.com/genpage.php?tname=nutrient&dbid=112 Retrieved on 7/28/18

[22] Cinnamon: https://www.healthline.com/nutrition/10-proven-benefits-of-cinnamon Retrieved on 9/20/18

[23] Calcium: https://draxe.com/foods-high-in-calcium/ Retrieved on 07-30-2018 * https://www.myfooddata.com/articles/foods-high-in-calcium.php Retrieved on 07-30-2018 * http://www.whfoods.com/genpage.php?tname=nutrient&dbid=45 Retrieved on 07-30-2018

[24] Vitamin D3 – Cholecalciferol: https://draxe.com/vitamin-d-deficiency-symptoms/ Retrieved on 7/28/18 * https://www.myfooddata.com/articles/high-vitamin-D-foods.php Retrieved on 7/28/18 * http://www.whfoods.com/genpage.php?tname=nutrient&dbid=110 Retrieved on 7/28/18

[25] Cod Liver Oil: https://nutritiondata.self.com/facts/fats-and-oils/628/2 Retrieved on 9/12/18

[26] Vitamin E: https://draxe.com/vitamin-e-foods/ Retrieved on 7/28/18 * https://www.myfooddata.com/articles/vitamin-e-foods.php Retrieved on 7/28/18 * http://www.whfoods.com/genpage.php?tname=nutrient&dbid=111 Retrieved on 7/28/18

[27] Potassium: http://draxe.com/low-potassium/ Retrieved on 8/23/18

[28] Low Sodium V-8: https://nutritiondata.self.com/facts/vegetables-and-vegetable-products/10452/2 Retrieved on 9/12/18

[29] Vinegar: https://www.healthline.com/nutrition/6-proven-health-benefits-of-apple-cider-vinegar Retrieved on 9/25/18

[30] Spirulina: https://nutritiondata.self.com/facts/vegetables-and-vegetable-products/2765/2 Retrieved on 9/12/18

[31] Clams: https://nutritiondata.self.com/facts/finfish-and-shellfish-products/4183/2 Retrieved on 9/12/18

[32] Iron: https://draxe.com/top-10-iron-rich-foods/ Retrieved on 7/30/18 * https://www.myfooddata.com/articles/food-sources-of-iron.php Retrieved on 7/30/18 * http://www.whfoods.com/genpage.php?tname=nutrient&dbid=70 Retrieved on 7/30/18

[33] Almonds: https://nutritiondata.self.com/facts/nut-and-seed-products/3087/2 Retrieved on 9/12/18

[34] Lentils: https://nutritiondata.self.com/facts/legumes-and-legume-products/4337/2 Retrieved on 9/12/18

[35] Chickpeas: https://nutritiondata.self.com/facts/legumes-and-legume-products/4325/2 Retrieved on 9/12/18

[36] Grapefruit: https://nutritiondata.self.com/facts/fruits-and-fruit-juices/1905/2 Retrieved on 9/12/18

[37] Olives and olive oil: http://www.whfoods.com/genpage.php?tname=foodspice&dbid=46 Retrieved on 9/18/18

[38] Phosphorus: https://draxe.com/foods-high-in-phosphorus/ Retrieved on 7/30/18 * https://www.myfooddata.com/articles/high-phosphorus-foods.php Retrieved on 7/30/18 * http://www.whfoods.com/genpage.php?tname=nutrient&dbid=127 Retrieved on 7/30/18

[39] Manganese: https://draxe.com/manganese/ Retrieved on 8/23/18

* https://www.myfooddata.com/articles/foods-high-in-manganese.php
Retrieved on 8/23/18

[40] Copper: https://draxe.com/foods-high-in-copper/ Retrieved on 8/23/18
* https://www.myfooddata.com/articles/high-copper-foods.php
Retrieved on 8/23/18 * http://www.whfoods.com/genpage.php?
tname=nutrient&dbid=53 Retrieved on 8/23/18

[41] Zinc: https://draxe.com/foods-high-in-zinc/ Retrieved on 8/23/18
* https://www.myfooddata.com/articles/high-zinc-foods.php Retrieved
on 8/23/18 * http://www.whfoods.com/genpage.php?tname=
nutrient&dbid=115 Retrieved on 8/23/18

[42] Chlorine: https://euromd.com/21-healthy-living/138-beauty-and-
fitness/4-vitamins-and-supplements/post-2300-why-body-needs-
chlorine/ Retrieved on 9/26/18

[43] Choline: https://draxe.com/what-is-choline/ Retrieved on 7/24/18
* http://www.whfoods.com/genpage.php?tname=nutrient&dbid=50
Retrieved on 7/24/18

[44] Bananas: https://nutritiondata.self.com/facts/fruits-and-fruit-
juices/1846/2 Retrieved on 9/12/18

[45] Turmeric: https://en.wikipedia.org/wiki/Curcumin Retrieved on 8/20/18

[46] Oregano: https://www.naturalfoodseries.com/9-health-benefits-
oregano/ Retrieved on 9/18/18

[47] Sage: https://www.webmd.com/vitamins/ai/ingredientmono-504/sage
Retrieved on 9/18/18

[49] Rosemary: http://www.whfoods.com/genpage.php?tname=
foodspice&dbid=75 Retrieved on 9/18/18

[50] Cloves: https://www.organicfacts.net/health-benefits/herbs-and-
spices/health-benefits-of-cloves.html Retrieved on 9/20/18

[51] Black pepper: https://draxe.com/peppercorns/ Retrieved on 9/12/18

[52] Paprika: https://draxe.com/paprika/ Retrieved on 9/25/18

[53] Vitamin A: https://draxe.com/top-10-vitamin-foods/ Retrieved on
7/23/18 * https://www.myfooddata.com/articles/food-sources-of-
vitamin-A.php Retrieved on 7/23/18 * http://www.whfoods.com/
genpage.php?tname=nutrient&dbid=106 Retrieved on 7/23/18

[54] Vitamin B1 – Thiamine: https://draxe.com/thiamine-foods/ Retrieved on
7/23/18 * https://ods.od.nih.gov/factsheets/Thiamin-HealthProfessional/
Retrieved on 7/23/18

[55] Vitamin B2 – Riboflavin: https://draxe.com/vitamin-b2/ Retrieved on
7/23/18 * http://www.whfoods.com/genpage.php?tname=nutrient&
dbid=93 Retrieved on 7/23/18 * https://www.myfooddata.com/articles/
foods-high-in-riboflavin-vitamin-B2.php Retrieved on 7/23/18 *
https://ods.od.nih.gov/factsheets/Riboflavin-HealthProfessional/
Retrieved on 7/23/18

[57] Vitamin B5 – Pantothenic acid: https://draxe.com/vitamin-b5/ Retrieved
on 7/24/18 * http://www.whfoods.com/genpage.php?tname=
nutrient&dbid=87 Retrieved on 7/24/18

[58] Vitamin B6 – Pyridoxine: https://draxe.com/top-10-vitamin-b6-foods/
Retrieved on 7/24/18 * http://www.whfoods.com/genpage.php?
tname=nutrient&dbid=108 Retrieved on 7/24/18

[59] Vitamin B7 – Biotin: https://draxe.com/biotin-benefits/ Retrieved on
7/24/18 * https://en.wikipedia.org/wiki/Biotin Retrieved on 7/24/18

[60] Vitamin B9 – Folate: https://draxe.com/top-10-vitamin-b9-folate-foods/
Retrieved on 7/24/18 * http://www.whfoods.com/
genpage.php?tname=nutrient&dbid=63 Retrieved on 7/24/18

[61] Vitamin B12 – Methylcobalamin: https://draxe.com/vitamin-b12/

benefits/ Retrieved on 7/24/18 * https://en.wikipedia.org/wiki/
Cobalamin Retrieved on 7/24/18

[62] Vitamin C: https://draxe.com/vitamin-c-benefits/ Retrieved on 7/26-18 *
https://www.myfooddata.com/articles/vitamin-c-foods.php Retrieved
on 7/26-18 * http://www.whfoods.com/genpage.php?tname=nutrient&
dbid=109 Retrieved on 7/26-18

[63] Molybdenum: http://www.whfoods.com/genpage.php?tname=nutrient
&dbid=128 Retrieved on 8/29-18

[64] Sulfur: https://en.wikipedia.org/wiki/Glucosinolate Retrieved on 8/20/18
* https://en.wikipedia.org/wiki/Isothiocyanate Retrieved on 8/20/18 *
https://en.wikipedia.org/wiki/Indoles Retrieved on 8/20/18

[65] Net Negative Calorie foods: https://nutritionfacts.org/18/06/07/foods-
with-negative-calories/ Retrieved on 9/18/18 * https://food.ndtv.com
/food-drinks/11-foods-that-burn-more-calories-than-they-contain-
1679965 Retrieved on 9/18/18 * https://en.wikipedia.org/wiki/
Negative-calorie_food Retrieved on 9/18/18

[66] ORAC Scores (for antioxidants): http://www.superfoodly.com
Retrieved on 8-29-18

[67] Chlorophyll: https://draxe.com/chlorophyll-benefits/ Retrieved on
8/20/18 * https://en.wikipedia.org/wiki/Chlorophyll Retrieved on
8/20/18

[68] Human liver: Lambert, Brent https://www.feelguide.com/2010/11/13/
did-you-know-the-regeneration-of-the-human-body-2/